ON HIPPOCRATES' ON THE NATURE OF MAN

Claudius Galen

Translated by: *W.J. Lewis*
Edited by: *D.P. Curtin*

Dalcassian
Publishing
Company
PHILADELPHIA, PA

On Hippocrates' On the Nature of Man

‘

Library of Congress Cataloging-in-Publication Data

On Hippocrates' On the Nature of Man

1-2. Some time ago, when I wrote a treatise, *Concerning the Elements According to Hippocrates*, and gave it to one of my friends who had been sent abroad, I oriented it towards his background. For as I knew he was already well-versed in this area, I did not present any proofs at the beginning of the treatise, nor did I give a review, as it is customary to do when a general argument is about to be presented to all those unfamiliar with it. With this work having been written first, I did not know how to draw from it for a general audience, nor did it seem advisable to write a second treatise. Moreover, I was reluctant to write a commentary on the book *On the Nature of Man*, because it clearly dealt with all the things covered by this treatise *Concerning the Elements According to Hippocrates*, which had already been published.

But now, since friends have asked me for a commentary on the Hippocratic treatise, *On the Nature of Man*, a commentary not only on the passages indispensable for the teaching of it, but on all the passages in turn, I will begin by first writing those things which I omitted to say at the beginning of the commentary *Concerning the Elements According to Hippocrates*, since I knew that my friend was already familiar with them.

2-5. There is one thing to address first: what, then, is meant by this word 'nature', from which some of the ancient philosophers were called 'natural' philosophers? This will become clear to those of you who are unfamiliar with these philosophers' books titled *On Nature*, those of you on whose account I am writing this. For it seems that these books are explaining what sort of thing the primary substance is: the substance which they say is the ungenerated cause underlying all generated and perishable bodies, existing by its own logic in each generated and perishable thing. The knowledge of other things which are not known by their own logic follows for each of the substances in turn, once these generated and perishable things are known. For a complete lesson on the nature of each existing thing takes place if someone explains one or two existing things in some detail, and men are accustomed to say that they explain about the nature of the situation to some extent, just as the Poet does; for he says (*Odyssey* 10.302-303):

As Hermes, having spoken clearly, furnished medicine, pulling it from the earth, and showed to me its nature.

And he says in turn that the root was black, and the blossom resembling milk. So, those who wrote about herbs, or about plants in general, taught about the observable nature of these plants (what qualities they have to someone touching, tasting, smelling or seeing them), and they claimed that some of them have a power either when taken into the body or applied to the outside. For the observable nature of each existing thing lies in these qualities. And of the ones above, it is the first nature concerning which I have spoken, and concerning which Plato advises us to be aware that someone who wishes to understand this should undertake the process methodically. I will include for you this passage of his (*Phaedrus* 270c3):

Do you think it is possible to understand the nature of the soul properly by reason, apart from the nature of the entire man?

If Hippocrates, of the Asclepiadian school, is to be trusted, the body cannot be understood except by this method.

He is correct, my friend. Still, it is necessary for us to examine logical reasoning with respect to Hippocrates, to see if it agrees.

All right.

What, then, does Hippocrates say that 'to observe concerning nature' is, and what does true reasoning say? For is it not necessary that the nature of anything whatsoever be understood in this way? First whether it is simple or complex. Then, if it is simple, to examine its power: what it possesses making it tend to act, and what tends to undergo its action. And if it has a complex form, then to examine it with respect to each individual aspect, in the same way that the simple was examined with respect to one aspect: what does it do by nature and what is affected by it.

This passage from Plato's *Phaedrus* teaches you the meaning of the term 'nature' and how it is necessary that its substance be studied methodically.

5-9. You may find all these things written in books titled *On Nature* by the ancient philosophers: Empedocles, Parmenides, Melissus, Alcmaeon, and Heraclitus. Some of them wrote not just one, but several books on this theory; some, like Epicurus, even wrote a great many. He begins as do all the others, with the question of whether there is one simple thing whose nature we are attempting to discover, or whether it is something constructed from some simple primaries of its own – 'elements', as those following the ancients were accustomed to call them. In the same way, with respect to speech, grammarians say that 'd' and 'k' are elements; that is, simple and primary parts which cannot be divided into others, as syllables can. For when you take the first element, sigma, from the syllable -stra-, you still have a syllable in the -tra- which remains. And so again, if you remove the first letter, -t-, from this -tra-, you will have -ra- left over from this, which can still be divided. However, you cannot divide the -a- and show it to be composed of two or three sounds, as many others are. For it is one indivisible sound in itself, not simply with respect to length, but with respect to form alone, as we and many other philosophers have shown elsewhere. So, those who say that the four elements of generated and perishable bodies are air, fire, earth and water, because none of them can be divided further into more forms, posit these as physiological primaries.

For, although the first concept of smallest bodies is based on size, the second, in turn, is based on quality, as is shown with elements of speech. And the natural philosophers disagreed with each other, some claiming that the elements are the smallest parts in generated and perishable bodies based on size, and some that they are the smallest based on quality. But in the first book of *On the Medical Terms*, the term 'element' is discussed at length, as is the term 'nature' in the fifth book. For now our argument concerns the practice itself, not terms or definitions. From these smallest elements (whether smallest with respect to size or to form), the first construction of generated bodies takes place, the bodies which Aristotle and I term "perceivable elements" and "uniformly composed materials." And from these there is another, second, synthesis of bodies which we call organs: the hand, leg, and eye, the tongue and lung and heart, and liver and spleen, kidneys, stomach, womb, and other such ones. For the primary nature of such organs relies on those primary and uniformly composed materials, which Plato was accustomed to call *protogona*. The difference between these bodies has also been discussed in a certain treatise, but the teaching, as far as the main points, will now be recounted clearly. Bone and cartilage and tendon are uniformly composed materials, as are membrane, fat and flesh; and that which joins to the sinews of muscles and to those uniform substances, and that which is in the viscera which Erasistratus calls *parenchuma*. And at the beginning of the study, *On the Therapeutic Method*, in which I explained what sort of thing this method is, it was shown that it is impossible to discover a treatment for uniform bodies without knowing whether each of them is simple, or is composed of many substances, and whether these are completely blended, or only touching each other. And it has been shown that some physicians, including Erasistratus, are half-way dogmatics, treating diseases of organs according to theory, but those of uniformly composed materials either empirically, or not entirely by theory. And most of them do not know how diseases of the organs differ from those arising in uniformly composed materials, just as they do not know the number of each of these. However, you, friends, have one of our treatises, *On the Differences of Diseases*, and a not insignificant procedure concerning remedies, which I have written as the *On The Therapeutic Method*. But both these and other things demand our opinion concerning the nature of the body, which will be taught in the present treatise.

9-11. So also, someone might marvel at those who think that the book *On the Nature of Man* is not one of the legitimate works of Hippocrates, but rather, as they are accustomed to say, a bastard work: they have been fooled by its arrangement, and by the interpolations in it; I will explain these things fully in this treatise. But for now it suffices to repeat what has been said in the treatise

On the Legitimate and Spurious Writings of Hippocrates, in the passage which reads thus:

The first part of the book from the letter A extends 240 lines, showing that the bodies of animals arise from hot and cold and dry and wet, and, after this, expounding on the nature of the humors. And what comes after this is varied. For the first part distinguishes those diseases called sporadic from the epidemics and plagues, and teaches the particular treatment for each kind in general. After that the work goes into the anatomy of blood vessels, and then there is a varied instruction on diseases. And after this, a healthy regimen for individual people is written about, and then, in turn, how someone can make stout people thin and thin people stout. And to this is joined instruction concerning emetics, and then a broad outline on the regimen of children and, after that, of women, and then of people who engage in exercise, and then finally it goes on for ten lines, apparently, about diseases of the brain, as it happens to be added. Thus it is very clear that the entire book is put together from many sources and is composed with an extent of barely 600 lines or a little less. It contains a first account, where it expounds concerning the elements and humors, in accordance with the system of Hippocrates, as well as a second account, where it expounds on the differences between epidemic and sporadic diseases. It also contains an appended work concerning the anatomy of blood vessels, which is completely spurious. For this appended work is not consistent with actual observation, and is at odds with what is said in the second book of the Epidemics. Although after this it sets down those topics which were investigated in the book which I have already written about, still these things are noteworthy, well-expressed and concise, and adhere to the system of Hippocrates, as do also those things which are said concerning the healthy regimen.

11-13. The complete book consists of these sections, but it is the first part of it which has as its foundation the entire system of Hippocrates. For this reason I have said that I am amazed that some people exclude this book from the thought of Hippocrates. Most of those who know the system of Hippocrates reckon this book with the legitimate works, considering it to be a writing by the great Hippocrates, although some think it is by Polybus, a pupil of Hippocrates, and also someone taking up the education of later generations, who seems to have altered none of the Hippocratic dogma at all in his own books, just as Thessalos, his son, did not. And Thessalos was a great man, but did not remain in his native land, as Polybus also did not. For he was a contemporary with Archelaus, king of Macedonia. So, as I have said, nearly all the other physicians, except for a certain few, believed the book *On the Nature of Man* to be by Hippocrates. Nor was Plato himself unacquainted with it. For indeed, in the *Phaedrus*, he writes this short passage, cited before, of which this is the beginning:

Do you think it is possible to understand the nature of the soul properly by reason, apart from the nature of the entire man?

On Hippocrates' On the Nature of Man

If Hippocrates, of the Asclepiadian school, is to be trusted, the body cannot be understood except by this method.

The people heedlessly talking nonsense, who are familiar with this passage, should investigate for themselves in which of the books by Hippocrates this method commended by Plato is written up. For besides the treatise we are now examining, *On the Nature of Man*, in no other does Hippocrates seem to investigate first concerning the human body – whether it is simple or complex – and then each of the other topics which Plato talked about, and which I have taught about in the *On the Elements According to Hippocrates*, and which we will nonetheless proceed to show, since this seemed good to you.

13-16. Having already gotten this far, I now come to the exegesis of the passages of this book by means of argumentations. Although my book, *On the Elements According to Hippocrates*, after it was made available to many people, was commended by every educated person, still, some uneducated people, who were unable to disprove any of the explanations in it, although they tried, were choked with jealousy, and they supposed that it would be sufficient slander to say that this work on which I was commenting is not by Hippocrates. But even if we were to grant that this work were not by Hippocrates or even by Polybus, and, if they wish, even grant that a certain work, *On the Nature of Man*, was not written with the first part demonstrating that our bodies are generated from hot and cold and dry and wet – even if we grant this to them, still, the idea that our bodies are generated and composed from these things is Hippocratic doctrine. For in the most well-known books of his, he seems to assume these origins, not only in considering the differences of diseases, but also thereafter in discovering the methods of curing. For diseases differ from each other with respect to hot and cold, wet and dry , and the treatment is to chill what is hot, and dry out what is wet; and similarly, to heat what is cold and make wet what is dry. Furthermore, he proposes that, of the natures pertaining to men before these diseases arise, some natures are hot, and some cold, some wet and some dry, and he supposes time and place to differ from each other in the same way, although Erasistratus says none of these things, nor does anyone else who supposes that what is hot is added on and not innate. In this way Hippocrates ascribes all the other things to these first principles point by point. But Erasistratus does not maintain this, and for this reason leaves some works on natural philosophy without an explanation, as we have said in the treatise *On the Natural Forces*. Since these people who slander everything proper complain about the length of the argument, or rather, say that I have written the entire treatise, I have decided to cut off this particular insult of theirs by writing a second work, in which I show the very doctrine of Hippocrates to whomever closely observes what is written in the *On the Nature of Man* and in all his other works. Again, I know that, regarding all the commentaries which I have written, the slanderers, ashamed to criticize works admired by everyone, instead cast blame on some of the observations made by people who agree with the works, as they are doing now. As for the books which have been written, they say that indeed Hippocrates made use of element-like objects (hot, cold, dry and wet), but that he did not truly accept this idea. And again when he explains that the body is composed of these things, they say that this work does not seem to be by Hippocrates, for they claim that the book *On the Nature of Man* is not by Hippocrates. As these people do not cease stirring up trouble, so you must remind them to remember what is set down in each of the treatises. And when we explain that Hippocrates, in all his writings, posited the foundation of his system in the knowledge of these discovered elements, they should not omit this when they investigate the truth, nor, when we investigate or explain the truth, should they draw back from consideration of his thought, but they should consider well for each thought whether the theory about the elements is true, and whether Hippocrates assumed these elements. So they should consider these two questions to begin with, both with reference to the *On the Elements According to Hippocrates* and with reference to the argument at hand. And from the abundance of what follows, it is apparent to those who are not stupid that the very one who wrote the book we have here is always postulating these same elements.

17.

Whoever is accustomed to hear people speaking about human nature beyond the extent to which it relates to medicine – it is not useful for him to hear this account. For I do not say that man is entirely air, or fire or water or earth or anything else which is not apparent as the one single thing existing in man; but I leave these things to those who wish to say them.

17-19. So far as this passage is concerned, it does not seem to be at all possible to learn clearly the intent of this work. For he censures those who take the account of nature further than what is useful for medicine: someone would conjecture that those carrying it further are the ones who say that the elements of the nature of man are fire and water and air and earth, and those who say it is a certain one of these elements: based on an immediate use of the imagination for the first opinion just mentioned, but according to careful examination for the second. And someone might expect that the ones who propose that our bodies arise from fire and earth and air and water mixed with each other would demonstrate that water or fire or earth or air are separated poorly in us, or, if not demonstrating this, would admit being refuted. For this is like expecting, with respect to the power of the medicine, *tetrapharmakon*, that one can demonstrate that it is pure wax or pitch or tallow or resin, or, if unable to demonstrate this, then not to grant that it is composed of these things. For in saying 'the four are blended' it is clear that there is no one of them which is pure. It is possible that it is meant either way in this present passage, but in what is said later, the second meaning seems to be intended by the writer. And if someone were to put his mind to it carefully, in the very passage where he says "*I do not say that man is entirely air*", he would not say that this means that there is no air in us at all, just as he does not mean that there is no fire or water or earth in us at all, but that we are not 'entirely' air. And the meaning of this phrase is 'not completely', not 'not at all'. For the matter concerning which we are writing is not completely negated by this phrase 'entirely', but its unmixed perfection is broken up. And indeed the Poet himself seems to be using this meaning for the word 'entirely' when he says (*Iliad* 13.349) "*He did not wish the Achaean people to be entirely destroyed beside Troy,*" and Hippocrates himself, when he says (*Aphorisms* 2.19) "*The prognoses of serious diseases are not entirely certain, neither of health nor of death.*" For the Poet is saying that Zeus, to oblige Thetis, desires to make a great slaughter of the Greeks, but not to utterly destroy them, and Hippocrates is saying that, although many prognoses are certain, as we have shown in our commentaries on the *Prognosticon*, not all of them are. So, as will be clear in its turn, it is best to take this phrase as meaning that Hippocrates does not agree with the ones who say that air is the only element of the human body, just as earth is not the only element, nor is water or fire. For it is not a certain one of these, but all elements.

20. Thus the phrase at the end of the passage, which is ambiguous in type with respect to distribution and combination, is better understood with reference to distribution, where he says "*nor some other thing which is not apparent as the one single thing existing in man.*" For this 'one single thing existing' (*hen eon*) is not, as the earlier exegetes supposed it to be, a single word, pronounced by the other Greeks in two syllables – *enon*, and in three syllables by the Ionians – *eneon*. Rather, it is two words: the one a monosyllable as when we are counting 'one (*hen*), two, three', the other as when we say 'existing' *(en)*, and the Ionians say *eon* with two syllables. For Hippocrates shows this in turn by arguing not against those who think the body consists of each of the four elements, but rather against those who think that the nature of man consists of a single one of these.

20-21. In what way, someone might ask, does this explanation, in which some people propose that the nature of man is some single element, go beyond medicine? Because, as the work will say a little later, it follows from this teaching that man never suffers. And one may also concede this: that it follows that there is one single cure. But there seem to be many kinds of ailments and many kinds of cures, so that this account is truly false.

21. We have already seen each of the things spoken of in these passages in turn, as he sets them forth.

For I say that man is not entirely air, nor entirely fire nor water nor earth.

21-24. Artemidorus, who also has the name Kapito, made an edition of the books of Hippocrates which was not only well-regarded by the emperor Hadrian, but even today is quite carefully studied by many people. So also did his contemporary Dioscorides. They both altered many things in transcribing the ancient writings which the exegetes of the Hippocratic books recognize as the only writings. And, in addition to many other things, Kapito altered the passage we have here, writing in this way: "*For I say that man is not entirely air, nor entirely fire nor water.*" For since he had found no book by an ancient author which holds that earth is the only element, nor, besides this, did he find such an explanation to have been proposed by the men, the Peripatetics, who had gathered together a certain recounting of this teaching, he boldly altered the text. It would have been better for this issue to have been evaluated as well by the people zealously investigating the question, to which man does the teaching about earth as the only element belong? For this is similar to asking, who thought it was advisable to bind the palm of the hand when it has been wounded, and who thought it good for the binding of the heel to be done otherwise than Hippocrates, and who the binding of the collar bone, or who binds a bone fracture accompanied by a wound not at the wound itself but on either side, or who, in cauterizing the shoulder joint, does not place the hot iron in the proper places, or who are the ones whom Hippocrates has criticized in his writing on the spine. For many such things are said by Hippocrates in the *On Fractures* and the *On Joints*, sometimes against one, sometimes against many mistaken people, just as in the *On the Acute Regimen*. And there, at the same time, he has written criticizing many physicians in these words (Littre 8.4):

I have seen physicians doing the opposite of what they ought. For at the beginning of the illness, they all impose on men a fast of two or three days, or more, and only then prescribe gruels and liquids.

Some of these physicians were the Regimenists, so the exegetes have shown us, and some were those who think man is phlegm alone, some were those who think he is yellow bile alone, and some black bile alone. Thereupon the exegetes who have taught thus said that some of these physicians were mentioned in this very book, *On the Nature of Man*. And it would have been better for the exegetes to say that not all of these physicians wrote down their own teachings in a timely manner. Indeed, it is possible that the writings of these physicians were not preserved. This happens for many reasons: some had no followers adopting their teaching, some did not publish books when they were alive, and then, after their death, the one or two remaining transcripts were lost. It is also possible that, because they were looked down on, their writings were neglected and in time finally lost. Some envious ones have hidden or obliterated the books of the ancients, and some have even done this so that they might say that the things written in these books are their own particular ideas. And who would be amazed that books by the writers of outlandish doctrines might have been destroyed, when even some comic and tragic poets who had won good reputations among the Athenians have been found to have no surviving dramas. That I may leave out all the other reasons, I will call to mind two alone, of those which have lately occurred in Rome: shrines having often burned and fallen down in earthquakes, or for some other reason having become causes of destruction for not a few books.

24-26. So Kapito was wrong in daring to alter the ancient passage, not allowing that it might be accepted that the first scribe was mistaken when he wrote one thing contradicting another. On the other hand, some of the exegetes have written falsely about Xenophanes, as Sabinus did when he included Xenophanes with these names.

For I do not say that man is entirely air, as Anaximenes does; nor fire, as Heraclitus; nor water, as Thales; nor earth, as a certain Xenophanes.

For nowhere is Xenophanes found clearly spoken of in this way. Rather, from this it is clear that Sabinus himself is speaking falsely about Xenophanes, and that he is not merely mistaken due to ignorance. Or, at any rate, he has added the name to the book in which these things are declared. For here he wrote thus: "...*nor earth, as a certain Xenophanes.*" But Theophrastus, in his summary of the teachings of natural philosophy, would have written about the doctrine of Xenophanes, if indeed he had one. And it is possible for you, if you enjoy this kind of research, to re-read the books of Theophrastes, in which he made a summary of the doctrine of natural philosophy, just as, in turn, if you wish to investigate the doctrines of the ancient physicians, you can re-read the books of the Medical Collection; these were ascribed to Aristotle, but are accepted as being by Menon, his student, for which reason some people call these books Menonian. For it is clear that this Menon carefully investigated the surviving books of ancient writers with respect to this topic and gathered their teachings. And it was impossible for him to record the ideas of those books which had already been lost, or which still survived but which he had not seen. So, in these books, you will not find even one person speak of yellow bile or black bile or phlegm as the element of the nature of man. But many of us, after Hippocrates, seem to think that blood, alone of these, is the element, since our first origin arises from it, and after this our growth in the womb and the conclusion of being born. But Hippocrates said a little later that there are some who consider man to be phlegm and bile, and he would not have written either for or against this idea if there were not some people conjecturing thus.

27-28.

But it seems to me that the ones who say these things do not understand correctly. Although they all make use of the same idea, yet they do not say the same things; rather they make the same epilogue to their ideas. For they say that there is one thing which exists and this is both the one single thing and everything, but they do not give it the same name. One of them says that air is this one single thing and everything, another says fire, another water, and another earth. And each adds to his account evidences and proofs which are nothing. For because they all use the same idea, but do not say the same things, it is clear that they do not understand. Someone who is present when they are debating may see this the most clearly. For the same men arguing against the same opponents never prevail three times in a row: first one is triumphant in his account, but then another prevails – whoever happens to have the most fluent tongue before the audience. Yet it is proper that the one who says he understands correctly should always have his own argument triumphant, if he understands what actually is, and explains it correctly. But these men clearly seem to me to overturn themselves in the words of their accounts through stupidity, and to confirm the theory of Melissus.

28-29. So, he makes an argument against what is said by those who propose a single element. For some, saying that fire is the element, would have it that the other elements arise from fire when it is packed together and compressed and compacted, with air being the least compression of it, water of a greater compression, and earth of the final and greatest compression. By the same argument, others say that water, and still others that air, gives rise to the other elements as they are compressed or dispersed. For they say compressed water produces earth, and dispersed water produces air, just as compressed air produces water, and dispersed air produces fire, so that from the change of these four into each other, this argument urges that a certain one of these is the element. And for this reason, he says they *"use the same idea, but do not say the same things."*

29-31. So, clearly, in this account he disagrees with all the ones who propose that one particular element of the four is man, and he says they are wrong. For because they demonstrated nothing, their argument was utterly unconvincing. They do not provide an argument that man is a certain one of the four elements, but, rather, they support the argument of Melissus, who claimed that there was a single element out of which man was made, but that it was not a particular one of these four, i.e. not air, earth, water or fire. And this man, Melissus, seems to have thought there was some common substance serving as a foundation for the four elements, an ungenerated and imperishable substance, which some after him called 'matter', but he seems to have been unable to make this clear in complete detail. Still, he says that this substance is the one single thing and also everything. But this account is not true. For this one certain something, the source of bodies in origin and destruction, as Melissus assumes, does not exist, but instead of this, there are four qualities, the extremes of coldness, dryness, heat and wetness. And indeed these are not the elements of the nature of man or of others, but of the first principles. This was confused by the ancients who had not yet conceived the idea of differences between 'first principle' and 'element', since they were able to use the term 'elements' for 'first principles'. But clearly the two things are different from each other: the one is the smallest part of a whole, while the other is that smallest thing which can be distinguished in thought. For fire is not able to divide into two bodies and to be shown to be a mixture of them, just as earth cannot, nor water, nor air. Indeed, it is possible to think that the substance belonging to the altering body is one thing, and its alteration is another thing. For an altering body is not the same thing as the alteration in it. The altering body is the underlying thing, and its alteration comes about in the change of its qualities. A body shows the extremes of inborn heat when a fire comes to be in it. Likewise when air comes to be, it shows the extreme of wetness. And in the same way when earth arises then the underlying thing, being originally featureless in itself, shows to all, in its own nature, dryness without heat, and when water arises it shows coldness. There has been no small investigation into this first cold thing, but its usefulness has no connection with the present discussion and the investigation has accomplished nothing in the medical arts. For the most useful thing in the investigation is whether the human body is one simple material, or a compound of four simple materials as the passage of Plato has taught, and as we have taught widely in the first part of the *On the Therapeutic Method*.

31-32. But this will be discussed again; and for now we will bear in mind that in this present passage he made an argument against those who say that man is one single element of the four, but not against those who say that man is four. Thus, in the first passage the better reading is naturally taken as a rough breathing at the onset of the first syllable of *hen eon*. For Hippocrates shows that it is not one single thing, but several, which underlie the nature of man; indeed none of the four elements exists in the body in a pure state. For the ones who assert this teaching do not say that this single element is the foundation. Rather, they declare that there is some single thing besides these four, composed of them, just as if the *Tetrapharmikon* curative force were not wax and pitch and resin and tallow, but some other single thing besides them, a thing which originated from a mixture of all these, so that this is an ambiguity. For some say that the four single qualities are mixed with each other completely, while others declare it is the substances which are mixed. The Peripatetics follow the first teaching, and the Stoics the second. Before them, Empedocles asserted that the nature of the body was constructed from the four unchanging elements, as from primary things mixed with each other, just as someone who has carefully emulsified and worked them into fine powder, would mix rust and bronze and cadmium and *misu* and so not be able to construct anything from any one of them without the other.

33.

Of the physicians, some say that man is blood, some that he is bile, and some phlegm.

In the argument on this subject, he has spoken against the philosophers who think that the nature of our body is fire alone, or water, or earth, or air, and in this passage he turns to physicians and shows that they have been similarly mistaken in these matters, those ones who think that man is either blood alone, or bile or phlegm. So it has already been clearly declared that the teaching in the very first passage is ambiguous: for he does not appear to argue against those who assume four elements, but always against those assuming one single element of the four. A certain teaching, analogous to that of Melissus, is omitted here, the teaching of physicians who say that man is a single substance which changes into each of the afore-mentioned elements.

34.

And they all make the same epilogue. For they say that it is one single thing, whatever each one wishes to call it, and this thing changes its form and power as it is constrained by hot and cold, and becomes sweet and bitter and white and black and so on. But these things seem to me not to be so.

34-35. And he says that the physicians who have said that there is one single humor in nature have made the same epilogue as each other and as the philosophers, when they declare that the one particular humor which each of them assumes, changes into the others. In constructing these arguments, each maintains his own teaching, nor do they show that only one of the four humors exists in nature, but that there is some humor first before the others, from which, when it is changed, these others are generated (such a fifth doctrine can be constructed concerning medical theory, analogous to that of Melissus concerning natural philosophy). These physicians, indeed, say that this one single thing changes, "*constrained by hot and cold, and becomes sweet and bitter and white and black*", and they do not seem to speak about the four humors, in contrast to the people he argued against when he said there was not this one single thing in nature. On the contrary, these physicians seem to say that something else is changing into these things. For blood is said to be sweet naturally, and yellow bile to be bitter, phlegm to be white, and black bile black, and they say that the one single thing changes into these as it is constrained by hot and cold.

35. This entire section at the end of the argument shows the ichors which arise in difficult illnesses. And, indeed, greenish bile and gray bile (they call this woad-ish) can be seen, as well as a certain red one and a grass-green one, and other nameless ones, especially when the disease is putrefying.

36.

But I say: if a man were one single thing he would never suffer, for there would be nothing from which he, as one single thing, could suffer; and if he did suffer, there would necessarily be a single treatment.

36-37. First he condemns the arguments given by those who claim that man is one single thing, showing that these accounts are not only unproved, but also unconvincing. With these arguments, he now refutes the teaching of those who think that man is one single thing. For it is not the same thing to argue against a proposed explanation, as it is to condemn a teaching as untrue. Indeed, he shows that the teaching is true, but not correctly argued by some people, and, in this way, the disagreement does not arise with the teaching, but with those arguing for it. Thus, now putting their explanations to one side, he argues against the very teaching alone, using not only the strongest argument against it, but also the shortest. For he says, "*If man were one single thing, he would never suffer.*" And he said that any explanation refutes those who assume that the smallest elements are indivisible and unjoined. For that which truly exists is one single thing, both in form and with respect to being indivisible and unjoined. And thus, the primary body is called ungenerated and indestructible, since all the others take their origin from its composition. For from these assumptions, the teaching has arisen which postulates that we have our origin in a kind of synthesis of these eternal bodies, as Hippocrates postulates, in the mixture of the four elements, which Aristotle and the Stoics assumed. And he says that the proof that, if there were one single element, the body composed of such an element would not suffer, is that no other, second element, able to act, is present in the body. For he does not grant that a single body in this situation would be affected on its own, and, even if someone were to grant that it, being affected, could suffer on its own, then there would be a single cure; for with there not being many illnesses in the body, it would be impossible for many types of cures to arise. But, in fact, there are many types of cures.

38.

There are many things existing in the body, which, when they are by nature heated, cooled, dried and made wet with respect to each other, bring forth diseases. And just as there are many individual ailments, so there are many treatments.

38-40. In the passage before this one, he completely refuted those who say man is one single thing, which is the same as saying that he is composed of one element, based on the strange implications of that teaching. For we would not suffer if there were no other, second element able to affect this first one. And even if we were to grant this, then there would be a single type of cure, not many types. In the passage we have here, he discusses these things which he will show as being primary, from which all the others originate. These are hot and cold and dry and wet. When these are mixed with each other in a well-balanced way, the creature is healthy; but when any one of them is heated and chilled, dried and made wet, it naturally produces ailments which are not cured by merely one method. For some ailments disappear when the afflicted parts have been heated, some when they have been chilled or dried or made wet. These things are discussed further in the writings *On the Power of Simple Medicines* and *On the Therapeutic Method*. And this is not a bad place now to say something short and clear containing a demonstration of our suffering through hot, cold, dry and wet, and our being cured. For who does not know that ailments occur, when someone goes outside in the excessively strong winter storms, and when someone goes out in excessive heat? Who does not suffer when they are thirsty or when they are completely filled with liquid – the thirst arising when we are dried, and the over-fullness causing the opposite condition? And inflammations, and all ailments and natural afflictions, sometimes arise from excessive wetness flowing into the body part, and sometimes from the humors being naturally hot, or cold. And indeed the cure for a body over-filled with wetness is accomplished by means of draining, and the cure for a body dried by nature is by the addition of wetness, just as the cure for one which has been heated is by chilling, and for one which has been chilled beyond what is appropriate, by means of heat. And all medicines are shown to be effective by means of heating or cooling or drying or making wet. For these are the vigorous and changing qualities of bodies, as we have shown in *On the Elements According to Hippocrates*. And the qualities of taste also correspond to these; the names of which are harshness, bitterness, astringency, sharpness, saltiness, pungency, acidity, sweetness, and oiliness; the qualities of color exist in white and black and red and those of the same origin; the qualities with respect to touch in hardness, softness, roughness, and slipperiness. The qualities of smell are equal in number to those of taste, but they do not have their own names. For the difference between a good smell and a bad one may properly be considered and spoken of in the same way as the difference corresponding to the many types of taste.

41. These are the main points of the argument. Some of them are demonstrated in the *On the Elements According to Hippocrates*, and some in the *On the Practice of Simple Medicines*. Many shrink from learning these explanations, and argue readily against things which they do not know. In contrast to this, those who love to learn and are lovers of truth work diligently, learning these explanations, and arguing against them only reluctantly.

But I expect someone who has said that man is blood alone, and nothing else, not to show that man changing his nature, nor becoming various, but rather to show that either in some season of the year or some time of a man's life, man seems to be one single thing alone, blood. For it is likely that there would be one time in which this blood appears on its own as the single thing existing. And I say the same thing concerning someone who says man is phlegm, and those who say he is bile.

42. And here he is still arguing against those who say that man is a single element, just as I have said that he proposed from the beginning. Firstly, he has criticized those who say that man is blood. He said that, if the nature of the body were blood alone, it must be the case, that healthy men would have blood alone in their bodies, without biles and phlegm, and, even if it were granted that at some time bile and phlegm might be present, then still a certain time of life or season of the year would be found in which blood alone would be in the body without the other humors. And in the same way he criticizes those who say that man is bile or phlegm, as if the particular element existed naturally alone; and he also criticizes those who assume in this way that the first origin arises from this particular humor.

42-43.
I myself will show that these things which I claim that man is, according to convention and to nature, are always the same and alike, in one who is young and one who is old, in the cold season and the hot; and I will bring evidence and set forth the necessary causes by which each thing increases and perishes in the body.

43. He announces that he will demonstrate completely that those elements which he assumes to be present in the body increase and perish (that is, decrease), maintaining a presence according to time of life and season. And 'according to convention' refers to that which is thought and taught by men as the ancients were accustomed to term it, and 'according to nature' to that which is thought based on the very truth of what occurs.

First of all, it is necessarily the case that generation does not arise from one single thing. For how could some single thing generate another, if it is not mixed with some other thing?

44-45. Hippocrates always follows the manifest evidence. For this reason, he says here that nothing is generated from one single thing without the need of some other external thing, and the need of this mixture being well-balanced. But some of the ones who are called natural philosophers did not know how to undertake the explanation of a strange teaching which overturned natural theory. For he who says that the one single thing is the essence, logically eliminates all generation. Indeed, if the one single thing is a generated thing, then it did not exist earlier, just as it will not exist a little later. For neither Thales nor Melissos nor Heraclitus existed at an earlier point, if they now exist. So, could someone truly say that these men were not generated? Or, is it that they were born and lived a number of years, each of them, but yet did not exist during the time they were alive? Or will we concede that they were there during this time, but say that they were not "existing", when they were? For indeed if someone agrees that they were existing, he agrees that they were generated. But how? And the plane tree, and the stone and the lion, which have an origin and a perishing, did they not exist long ago? Or, if there is an origin of something which did not exist at first, it is necessary that this origin arise from some underlying substance. And we see that this origin can not arise at all with reference to the same single substance. Indeed, the seeds of plants require wetness and heat from the outside in proportion, in order to be generated in some way. For if a seed were naturally capable of generating by itself, needing nothing else from the outside, then it would not wait even the shortest time without generating, but would immediately grow. But not a few seeds often seem to wait not merely a single month, but even a year. For they are not able to generate merely from themselves, but they require some external assistance which does not occur in the single grain, but in the power of something which touches it, and this external assistance is distributed inside, in the entire thing which is touched. And if it generally appears that this externally triggered alteration prevails over the seed in these origins where trees and grasses and plants in general are concerned, all the more clearly does it appear that in animals something cannot be generated from the male alone, or from the female alone, without some mixture.

46.
Then, if those which are not of the same kind and having the same power, should mate, there would be no generation, nor would we have these ones reproducing.

He says that not only is it impossible for something to be generated from a single source, but also not even from two, "*if those not of the same kind ... should mate,*" that is, those not possessing a kinship with respect to substance. And these things are clearly seen occurring in the generation of heterogeneous animals, as happens with horses and asses, and with foxes and dogs. For from the union of these, a certain type of animal is generated such that it is a mixture of both species, but these animals possess a nature which greatly stands out from the others, and, if they mate, they are unable to generate anything.

46-47. The exegetes of this book have passed by the phrase at the end of this passage, "*nor would we have these ones reproducing*", as if it were clear, but it is, in fact, unclear whether this has not been explained well by the writer or whether there has been a mistake by the transcribers. But it seems to me that what he wants to make clear is this: he says that if one animal should mate with another of a different type, there must be some sort of shared nature or "*we would not have these ones reproducing*", that is, no generation would arise from the union with an animal merely similar in origin. But perhaps, also, this passage is not genuine:

nor would we have these ones reproducing... (47) And if heat and cold do not occur equally and proportionately to one another, and dryness and wetness, but one dominates the other, the stronger dominating the weaker, then generation does not take place.

47-49. He said earlier that no fruitful generation can be accomplished, if the uniting parties are not of the same kind. Now he adds that the union even of those of the same type does not necessarily generate offspring. This last view of his can be read in the *Aphorisms*, where he says (5.62),

The ones who have cold stiff wombs, will not become pregnant. And those with excessively wet wombs will not become pregnant; for the offspring is extinguished. Also, the ones with dry and excessively heated wombs will not become pregnant, for the seed perishes due to lack of nourishment. But as for the ones with a well-proportioned mixture of both wetness and dryness, they will become pregnant.

In this discussion, he teaches that women become infertile for certain reasons, and he also points out what follows closely on this, concerning which we have written elsewhere, and many others besides us. Plato, as well, has made this clear, saying that it is no insignificant skill, by which someone may know that men and women possessing a similar combination may unite in generation. For he says these things concerning the balance in the womb, and one must also bear these in mind with respect to the seed. For this, also, is sometimes more wet than is needed, or more cold, and sometimes dryer and more heated. For a wetter seed is appropriate to a dryer womb, and a dryer seed to a wetter womb, just as also a colder seed to a hotter womb, and a hotter seed to a colder womb. We go into these matters further in the work on generation. For now it suffices to know that it is not possible for something to be generated from a single source, nor, when it is generated from two, or even more, uniting parties, can it be generated, without a certain well-balanced combination brought forth by the uniting partners being appropriate to each other.

49.
How is it likely for something to be generated from one source, when it is not even generated from many, if it does not happen that they possess a combination well-suited to each other?

49-50. The rest of this passage is clear from what has been said already, but it is necessary to bear in mind this term "combination" (*krasis*) used in it, which he expresses with the form *kresis*, because Hippocrates was the first of those we know to propose that the elements are combined, as was shown a little earlier, and he differed from Empedocles in this. For Empedocles says that we, and all the other earthly bodies, are generated from the same elements assumed by Hippocrates, and these elements are not combined with each other, but, as small pieces, stand next to each other, touching. It is made clear in the treatise, *On the Elements According to Hippocrates*, where we review nearly all the opinions about nature which have arisen concerning the first principles and elements, that this teaching of Empedocles already has the same refutations which were made against the teachings which assume a sensate body generated from insensate and unfeeling first bodies.

50.

Such being the nature of man and of all others, it is necessarily the case that man is not a single thing, but rather, that each of the things coming together in the generation possesses in the body a certain power, of the sort which it contributes.

51-53. Having said that, if heat is not mixed proportionately to cold, and dryness to wetness, it is impossible for the generation of generated bodies to occur, now Hippocrates says clearly that the generation, not only of man but of everything, is from those things which control the generation and perishing of bodies: that all things are generated from heat, cold, dryness and wetness, and for this reason these elements are common to all. Blood, phlegm, yellow bile and black bile are the particular elements of the nature of man. And yet, these things might not be properly called 'particular', for they are common to all animals with blood. And it is quite clear that each of them comes from the four primary elements which we call wetness, dryness, cold and heat, naming them after their qualities; the specific terms fire, water, air, and earth are from their substance. For it is clear that the elements are named with respect to simple unmixed qualities: the extreme heat being in fire, as extreme wetness is in air, coldness in water, and extreme dryness, along with compression and cold, in reference to earth. Thus, how can some people think that Hippocrates assumed that wetness, dryness, cold and heat were the elements (for these appear in man), but did not accept fire, water, air and earth (since some of these do not appear in the human body)? Indeed, they are not following their own logic, because if we were to say that these things apparent in the case of the body – the hot things, the cold things, the dry, the wet – are elements common to all bodies; by this logic a stone and each animate and inanimate body would be blood and phlegm and the two biles, as indeed they would be bone and cartilage and veins and arteries and sinew and all the things apparent in the body which are hot and cold, dry and wet. But who would dare to say these are elements common to all bodies? Not even the most dull-witted, since Hippocrates has said: "*so it is necessarily the case that there be such a nature of man and of all the others.*" It must be that he did not intend to say that heat, cold, dryness and wetness were visible things in the human body, but that they were the four elements. And they possess the unmixed, extreme quality from which, once they are combined with each other, all the intermediate bodies come into force; bodies, which, to be precise, should not be termed hot, cold, dry and wet. For if we assume that these things which are already combined are the elements, then I do not know what things we would say possess the extreme qualities. And in this passage here he shows most clearly his own opinion, to which we have already referred.

53.

And again, it is necessarily the case that, when a man's body dies, each element of it returns into its own nature: wet to wet, dry to dry, hot to hot, and cold to cold.

On Hippocrates' On the Nature of Man

53-54. He says that when a man dies, each one of the afore-mentioned separate elements returns to its own nature; and he calls these elements hot, cold, dry, and wet. Indeed, he does not say that blood returns to some cosmic blood, and phlegm to phlegm, bile to bile, artery to artery, flesh to flesh, vein to vein and sinew to sinew, but that in each of these, hot and cold and wetness and dryness returns to the elements common to all. For indeed the sinew consists of heat, cold, dryness and wetness; of the elements, that is. For it does not consist of another sinew, just as a vein does not consist of another vein, since it cannot be imagined that these are mixed from each other entirely: flesh and vein and bone and artery and the other parts. He maintains that hot, cold, dry and wet are generally mixed with each other, if we recall what was said a little earlier. So the hot, cold, dry and wet parts seen clearly in the human body, are not the elements of the nature of man, but compositions and generations of these elements; water, fire, air, and earth. And there is ample discussion of these matters in *On the Elements According to Hippocrates*.

55. "*Such also is the nature of animals and all others.*"

55-57. Such, he says, is not only the nature of man, but of all others, that is, a nature combined of the simple extremes of hot, cold, dry and wet. All the intermediate components contain the combination of these extremes. Thus it becomes unimaginable to say that the combination of these intermediate elements is generated from intermediate elements. For the ones who say that our nature is composed of the observable wet, dry, hot, and cold parts in the body do not understand the matter. It is even more inconceivable, if we say that the nature of all other animals and plants is from these intermediate components. For Hippocrates said clearly in this passage that "*all the others*" have the same nature. But these other people, however, do not know what they say. Indeed, after a fig-tree seed is sown in the earth, if it should happen that it generates a great tree, it is inconceivable to say that this substance arose, not from earth and water, but from some other thing in itself. And earth, according to its own manner, is cold in the extreme, but the fig-tree has a great deal of heat, by which it lives, and on this account, even when it is chilled in winter storms, it does not die. Thus it is clear that the body of the fig-tree does not consist only of earth and water, but that it has a share in the fiery nature, and it is obvious that it also has a share in the aerial nature, since indeed its wood is not only of earth, but also lighter than water. Thus the fig-tree is made of the four elements. And if it is, so is the fig. And so are all fruits (and wheat, barley, beans, and the rest of Demeter's seeds are parts of fruits); these are made from the four – earth, fire, water, and air. And then the humors, in turn, arise in us out of the food of the fruit and plants, and these clearly possess the first principle of generation: water, earth, air and fire. But, since, as I have said, these things are explained in the *On the Elements According to Hippocrates*, now it is the proper time to turn to the next passage.

57. "*These all arise similarly and come to an end similarly.*"

A person who supposed that there would be some men who might misunderstand him, would not repeat this same thought as many times as Hippocrates does now when he says that not only man, but all things, are generated and perish similarly, as has been said, from these four, namely the elements, not from the hot or cold or dry or wet parts of the body. But some people are not aware of the Greek reading, so that they suppose that the hot, cold, wetness and dryness in the human body as they are clearly observed by all, are the common elements of generation.

58.
For their nature consists of all these afore-mentioned things, and each thing ends, according to what has been said, in that same situation from which it arose. And thus it retreats there.

He continues with this thought, saying that the nature of all things consists of the four mentioned above, and that it ends in the same four. Whence each existing thing arises, he says, thence it returns: into the common elements of the cosmos, namely earth, water, air and fire. So they are extremely unfamiliar with Hippocratic opinion, the ones who take what was said at the beginning, "*for I say man is not entirely air nor water nor fire nor earth*", as equivalent to "*man is not at all...*" For Hippocrates did not say that the elements common to all were "*not at all*" in the human body, but rather, he was disagreeing with those who say that the nature of man is one single element of those in the body.

59.
The human body has in itself blood and phlegm and yellow bile and black bile, and this is the nature of the body, and through these it ails and is healthy.

59-60. Having completed his explanation of the common elements with reference to living creatures, of which man is one, he goes on with this present passage, saying from the beginning that our origin arises from blood and phlegm and both biles, and that permanence during the entire life is maintained from these elements, and that they are the nature of man on the one hand, because the humors surround solid things, and on the other because the solid things possess an origin from these elements in the first shaping of the fetus. For out of the menstrual material all the parts are born, not from pure blood, but from blood which possesses in itself both biles, and phlegm. And he will show this a little later. Indeed, he also says, in this passage we have here, that our being healthy, and our ailing and being sick come about from the nature of these elements, and the manner by which they arise.

60.

So the body is most healthy, when it has these elements in balanced proportion to each other, with respect to force and to amount, and especially if they are mixed.

60-61. According to all physicians, and the accomplished dogmatic philosophers, a good balance of the elements produces health. But the theory of elements in the schools of logic can be taken in two ways with respect to birth: one school says that the generation of compounds arises in a juxtaposition and intertwining of primary bodies; the other that it arises in a combined form. The first theory assumes a proper proportion in the porousness while the second theory, of which Hippocrates was clearly the chief proponent, assumes that our nature is healthy with respect to a balanced mixture of elements. Since 'proper proportion' is ambiguous, defined on the one hand by the force of the things which are mixed, and on the other by the amount of the substance, Hippocrates bears both aspects in mind, saying "*with respect to force and to amount*".

61. The phrase "*and especially if they are mixed,*" at the end of the passage, demonstrates the perfection of the mixture throughout the whole. In a completely perfect composition of the body, not only the proper proportion of the four elements, but also the mixture throughout the whole, is perfected. With respect to the more common mixtures of the body, it is shown that at some times in some single part the humors are mixed with each other neither equally nor similarly throughout the whole. And even when the function has clearly not yet deteriorated, still the health is compromised, although there is not yet any illness.

It feels pain when one of these becomes lesser or greater or is isolated in the body and not mixed with the others.

62. Just as he proposed that, in health, there is an exact proper proportion in amount and force and the mixture throughout the whole, so, in the same way he proposed the opposite of this for illness, referring on the one hand to something lesser or greater with respect to the amount of substance or with respect to force, and on the other hand, to it being mixed with things in a poorly balanced mixture, or in an irregularity of mixture, or whatever someone may want to call it.

It is necessarily the case that when one of these is isolated or stands by itself, not only will that place which it has left become diseased, but that place where it now stands and flows into will also be troubled and in pain because of being overfull.

62-63. When one of the four elements stands by itself somehow, isolated from the others in one part, and is whole, not being mixed with these in entirety, the creature suffers due to the poor balance which has come about in both parts: the place which the humor has left and the one into which it has gone. And this happens in particular with the humors which possess strong powers. For these not only oppress the part in which they now stand by their quantity, but they also produce pain by their quality: either heating or chilling excessively.

63.

For also, when one of these flows out of the body more than is prevalent at the surface, the draining causes pain.

One must understand that the "*more than is prevalent at the surface*" is said in place of "*more than the excess*", or, if someone does not want to take it this way, it must be understood to mean that "*that which is prevalent at the surface*" is that which has not mixed with all the others. For either interpretation is plausible.

63-64.

But if it should make a draining internally and a shifting and a separation from the others, it is quite necessarily the case that it will cause a double pain according to what has been said: in the place it has left and in the place to which it has overflowed.

64. He himself, by saying "*according to what has been said*" shows that he has already said this. For by this phrase, and not by the force of the present passage, what has been written by him a little earlier holds: where he says

It is necessarily the case that when one of these is separated and stands on its own, not only will that place which it has left become diseased, but that place where it now stands and flows into will also be troubled and in pain because of being overfull.

I have said that I will show that these things, the ones which I will say that man to be, remain the same always, according to both convention and nature.

He says "*according to convention*", intending that the teaching which people maintain about these things should be made clear, and "*according to nature*" that the truth of the practices themselves should be made clear.

65. Let us now turn our minds to the next passage in order to know if he will now return to that which he supported at the beginning of the treatise.

I say that these are blood and phlegm and yellow bile and black. First of all I say that the names of these are distinct according to convention, and that none of them share the same name; then I say that their particular characters are distinguished by nature, and phlegm does not at all resemble blood, nor blood resemble bile, nor bile resemble phlegm. How could these resemble each other, given that when they are seen they do not appear to be similar in color, nor when touched, do they seem similar to the hand? For they are not similarly hot nor cold nor dry nor wet.

65-66. His entire account is clear, and he demonstrates what he has proposed. For the previous passage showed that there are four humors in the body, differing from each other, and in the next passage, that these all exist by , not just one of them. But in this preceding passage he says that the humors differ from each other in color and structure and heat and cold and wetness and dryness. And these things are shown clearly.

66-67. Someone might object to the idea that one humor differs from another in dryness since all the humors are liquid. They should then take up the idea of humors not differing with respect to wetness. For if they suppose one of them to be more wet than another, they are obligated to suppose that the less wet one is such because of a mixture of the dry element. And indeed this is seen clearly with all the humors. For yellow bile is sometimes extremely liquidy, so that its color becomes not yellow, but pale, but sometimes thick like an egg-yolk, on which account it is called yolk-like by some. Black bile, in turn, is always thicker than the pale or yellow bile. And in black bile, the difference between the greater thickness and the lesser is not slight, just as is the case with blood. For blood also sometimes appears to be so liquid-like that it flows, but sometimes extremely thick. Phlegm, since it has the same relation, is included among the afore-mentioned humors. For it changes in thickness and lightness, sometimes being like water and sometimes thickened so that it is like pus. This fits in with the idea that the humors are not truly elements, as are water and earth, air and fire. For each of them is born of those four, one mixed with another of them, as you have often been instructed.

67.
When these differ so from each other with respect to shape and force, it is necessarily the case that they are not the same one, just as fire and water are not the same one.

67-69. And although the teaching of those who argue that man is one element is outlandish, still Hippocrates, in arguing against it, has made this clear with a zeal as great as that of the men famous for arguing against him, as they honored this very teaching. For since most of the writings of ancient men were not preserved, it is all the more unlikely that their unwritten teachings would be preserved, and especially because some of them wrote no treatises, like Socrates and Pythagoras and, of those physicians of high esteem in our own times, Quintus. Still more must it be believed that many men become famous while they are alive, and that then when they have died, the concepts of their thought are lost. Sometimes even the students of Plato, who did write such treatises, say that in addition to his writings there are some unwritten ideas of his. And just as we believe the students when they say that there are unwritten ideas, so also we trust that Hippocrates had access to some teachings which held that earth alone was the element common to all, and in man, bile or phlegm. For one now knows that there were some writers of strange things, whose treatises have already died with them, and have perished, just as the treatise by someone claiming that the mother and nurse and origin and element is the earth. She gave birth to the sky, as Hesiod says, and to the living creatures on her. One of the Archigenians, also, not the most worthless of men, believed that air did not enter the body in inhalations, nor exit in exhalations. And someone else proposed that the primary and elemental humor was phlegm. We will not seek the names of those who first proposed these strange teachings, given indeed that we are not even able to show from his writings that Thales declared that water was the only element, but this can be trusted in a similar way for all of them.

60-70.

You may know from these things, that these are not all one, but that each has its own force and nature. For if you were to give to a man a medicine which draws phlegm, he will vomit phlegm for you, and if you give him one which draws bile, he will vomit bile for you. In the same way, black bile is purged if you give a medicine which draws black bile, and if you cut a part of someone's body, so that a wound is made, his blood will flow. And all these things will happen for you every day and night, in winter and in summer, as long as he is still able to draw breath into himself and breathe it back out, or until he lacks one of the elements born into him. The afore-mentioned elements are born into him – how could they not be? First, a man clearly is seen to have in him all these elements, as long as he lives, and then, he is born from a human possessing all these, and then he is nourished in a human possessing all these – which I have said and demonstrated.

70-72. In the first passage Hippocrates clearly and truly showed that "*man entirely*" possesses all these things in himself: biles and phlegm and blood. And in this present passage he shows not only this, but that "*he possesses all these things*" by nature, not just one of them, as some say. But although the other opinions of those who say that there is one humor in the body by nature are easily refuted, the opinion of those who say it is blood is not easy to despise, but, rather, a great contest is necessary in order to reject this opinion. And it is now appropriate to establish the foundation from what was said earlier with respect to men, and also to establish the ones who did this. He says how in this way,

But I myself expect that someone who says that man is blood alone and nothing else, not to show that man changing his nature, nor becoming various, but rather to show that either in some season of the year or some time of a man's life man seems to be one single thing alone, blood. For it is likely that there would be one time in which this blood appears on its own as the single thing existing.

And if you add to this account what is shown in this present passage, you will reconstruct the thought of Hippocrates. For here he has shown that there is no single season and no such time of life in which someone can point to a man not having a share of all the humors, "*not only through common drainings*", but also through purges. And if you give to someone a medicine which draws out bile or phlegm you will see the drained matter drawn out according to its nature, since all things are present in the body in every season.

72-74. Some people disagree with this account, not conceding that an emetic draws its related humor out of the body, but claiming instead that the drained matter changes into that form which is the same by nature (i.e. into the related humor). However the fact that this account is false is demonstrated to you in the treatise *On the Power of Emetic Medicines*. And now, for the sake of argument, let one of the matters covered in this account be told. For in these works on the medical art you have seen people not infrequently denying that the drained matter was drawn out by the emetic medicines. In such a way, when those who are dropsical, of the type termed *askite*, have taken a medicine which draws out water, a quantity of watery liquid which is not insignificant is drained out and the size of the stomach is drawn in. But if someone should give them medicine which draws out yellow or black bile, it will draw out a very small amount of this humor and the size of the stomach will not only not become smaller, but will even become larger. On the other hand, you have seen the opposite results with those who suffer from a blockage of the liver. After their internal organs are unblocked by medicines which are capable of doing this, when the bile-drawing medicine is given, there is a great drainage of the overabundant humor and the pain immediately ceases. Note that something similar to this happens with respect to those suffering from phlegm or black bile. For the offending humor is drained in large quantity, and those who are suffering are greatly relieved. Accordingly, seeing that such things are drawn from the body by emetic medicines, and that these medicines purge at every time of life and season, then the four humors do exist continually in the human body. For it must be, as was said earlier, that at some one season of the year or time of a man's life, he would be seen possessing blood alone, if the opinion of those who claim that blood alone is the nature of man is assumed to be true; this is the same thing as all of his parts being made of blood alone and continually nourished by blood alone. But 'blood' is defined in two ways: on the one hand, as that which appears to be drained in blood-lettings and wounds, containing, as we have shown, both biles and phlegm; on the other hand, as blood pure and completely unmixed with any of the other humors. And it is probably true that a creature is formed from blood according to the first definition, but it is not true according to second definition. For this humor never appears alone in pregnant women. I think you know why I have added this to the account. For in the treatise *On Seed*, it was shown that most parts of the body arise from seed, with the fleshy parts alone formed from blood. But since the size of the seed deposited in the womb is small, its nourishment and increase comes about from blood, on account of which someone might almost say that parts are made of blood. For as much as the seed has its origin from blood, to that extent, someone who says that the origin of the fetus is from blood seems to be speaking truly, but it is not from pure blood, unmixed with the other humors, but from blood which is defined as a mixture.

75. Such is the entire intention of the passage here. And the first thing to be shown relating to it is the common habit not only of physicians, but of all Greeks, of naming bile without an epithet when they wish to refer to pale or yellow bile. I have said a little earlier that both these terms (i.e. 'pale' and 'yellow') are applied to one form of humor which varies in wetness and dryness. But they name all the other biles with an epithet, calling them either rust-colored or black or red or grass-green. And the second thing to be shown relates to this passage he says here: "*As long as he has the power to draw breath into himself and exhale again.*" For it is clear that he means when the inhalation of the respiratory organs drawing air from the outside takes place, and also the exhalation of the organs breathing out. And the third, where he says "*he lacks one of the elements born into him.*" For he means not only that, when he lacks blood, the creature dies, but also when he lacks phlegm or yellow or black bile.

76.

Those who say that man is one element seem to me to be using this idea: since they have seen those who drink drugs die in excessive purgings, some vomiting phlegm and some bile, they then suppose that man is whatever individual element of these, which they saw him die in trying to purge. And those who say that man is blood make use of the same idea. For, since they have seen men with their throats cut, and the blood flowing from the body, they suppose it to be the soul of man. And they all make use of such evidence in their arguments.

76-77. He says "*those who say man is one element*", since there are many who say this, not just one. Some of these people, thinking that a certain one of the four elements is sufficient to generate man, have persuaded themselves thus, not convincing us, but clearly convincing others, as Hippocrates himself has made clear. For, in these excessive purgings, because one of them sees a person die finally from one humor being purged, and another sees someone else die from the purging of another humor, they suppose that particular humor alone is the nature of man.

77.

And yet, first, in these excessive purgings no one has died somehow purging only bile, but when someone drinks medicine which draws out bile, first he vomits bile, and then phlegm and then after these, those who are pressed also vomit black bile, and finally pure blood.

77-78. And here again the custom of the Greeks is clearly shown: often naming yellow bile without an epithet, but always naming black bile with an epithet. This is clearly shown in the whole passage. For he says no one dies purging only bile, since the other humors are always purged with it.

78.

They suffer the same effects from medicines which draw out phlegm. First they vomit phlegm, then yellow bile, then black, and finally pure blood, after which they die.

After the humor particularly associated with the purging medicine is drained, then the most easily drawn out of the rest follows immediately after it in turn, and after that, the one having the second place to it, and then blood last of all, since it is the humor most related to the nature of man. For it is safe to say this concerning the matter: that even if the nature of man is not one single thing, still, of all the others, blood is the most related to it.

79.

For medicine, when it has entered the body, draws that first, which, of those things in the body, is most like it by nature, and then it draws and purges the others, just as plants and sown seeds, when they enter the earth, draw each thing in the earth most like themselves by nature. And these are sour and sweet and bitter and salty and all the rest. It draws to itself first that which is most related to it by nature, and then it draws the others. Medicines in the body also behave in such a manner. The ones which draw bile, first draw the purest, and then the mixed; and the medicines drawing phlegm draw the purest phlegm first and then the mixed, and for those who have been cut open, the blood first flows hottest and reddest, and then flows more phlegm-ish and bile-ish.

80. The passage clearly is by someone who wrote proofs of the present account, in which he says that medicine, when it has entered the body, first draws that humor most related to it, and then the others. It is necessary to bear in mind, with regard to plants, that he says that these draw into themselves each thing most like them by nature. For in the earth are sour and sweet and bitter and salty and all such. So clearly in man black bile is sour, yellow is bitter, blood is sweet and phlegm salty. In fact, phlegm is such that at one time it is sweet, at another sour, and at another without any distinguishing quality. On this account, it seems to me that he says "*and all such*" at the end of the passage, observing the various differences not only in phlegm, but also in the other humors. For just as sour, sweet, bitter and salty, so also there is an astringent and a harsh and an acrid and an oily form of humors in animals and plants and this is clearly comparable to those qualities in the earth.

81.

Phlegm increases in man in winter. For, of the things in the body, this is the most like winter by nature, since it is coldest. And the proof that it is the coldest is that, if you are to touch phlegm and bile and blood, you will find phlegm to be the coldest. And it is the most viscous, and, after black bile, requires the most force to draw. And whatever is drawn with force, becomes hotter under the pressure of that force. But, in spite of all these things phlegm appears to be coldest by its own nature. That winter fills the body with phlegm you may know by these observations: men spit and cough up the most phlegm-ish matter in the winter and their swellings become particularly white in this season and the other diseases become more phlegm-ish.

82. This entire passage is clear and demands that someone recognize and heed it, not that they explain it by exegesis.

And some people make an exegesis of the phrase "*and the other diseases become more phlegm-ish*" at the end of the passage, reading it without the article (i.e. "*and other phlegm-ish diseases arise*"). And swellings become more white in this season and more plentiful, and in this same season other diseases also become phlegm-ish; this is the meaning of the sentence if it is read with the article. Swellings become more white in the winter and the other diseases become phlegm-ish also at this time. And, of course, fevers , just as they are more bile-ish in the summer, so are more phlegm-ish in the winter.

And in spring, phlegm remains strong in the body and the blood increases. For the cold eases and the rains arrive, and the blood in these circumstances increases due to the rain showers and hot days. For by nature this time of year is most related to blood, since it is wet and hot. And you may know this by these observations: men in spring and summer are most likely to be stricken with dysentery, and blood flows from their noses and this blood is the hottest and reddest.

83-84. The meaning of this passage is clear. For it was said in the beginning of the *On Mixtures*, that spring is better described as a balanced mixture, not as wet and hot, and for this reason, some physicians and philosophers are reluctant to term this season hot and wet. But just as among the seasons they say this is wet and hot, so among the bodies of generated things, animals are wet and hot compared to plants, and spring, compared to the fall, is the best among the seasons, and, as someone might say, the only one holding itself strictly according to its nature, rather than incidental to its nature. And when the blood becomes full in the spring, along with other signs, then the afore-mentioned dysenteries clearly become bloody, but are not such as wound the bowels due to bile. For I have written concerning this bloody dysentery in the fourth book in the treatise *On Joints* which showed the affliction of an abundance of blood in the blood vessels which then often becomes a massing together of the nature which is excreted through the bowels, just as for women it is excreted through the womb, and for some people through their nose or hemorrhoids or vomiting.

84. And summer exceeds spring, based on the evidence of both dysenteries and the redness of the skin. For through its own heat the blood generated in the spring makes the skin of the entire body red, and for some people it is excreted through the anus. And men seem hot to those touching them at that time, on account of the blood and also on account of the surroundings.

84-85.

In summer blood is still strong, and bile rises in the body and extends into the autumn. And in the autumn blood becomes less, for autumn is opposite to it in nature. Bile dominates the body in summer and in fall. You may know this by these things: in this season men vomit bile on their own accord, and as for those taking purging-medicines, they purge the most bile-ish matter. This is also clear in the fevers and complexions of men. But in summer phlegm is weaker on its own account. For that season is opposite to it in nature, since it is dry and hot.

85. In the summer and especially at the beginning, for most people the blood, having increased in the spring, is plentiful, so that it is not yet carried off by the heat of the surroundings. And bile increases in this season on account of the body heating up naturally. And here again he uses the term 'bile' without appending the color-term 'yellow'; he never refers to black bile with the simple term alone, but always with the addition of the color-term. The points in this passage are clear step by step to those who are paying attention.

And blood in the autumn becomes least in man. For the autumn is dry and is already starting to chill man. But black bile is strongest and most plentiful in the autumn.

86. In this passage he says that in the autumn the blood becomes less. For the autumn is opposite to it by nature. And we have taught how it is opposite. For if the blood is wet and hot, like spring, and the autumn, as he himself says is "*dry and already begins to chill man*", then likewise autumn is opposite to spring and possesses most plentifully that humor, the dry and cold one, which is opposite to blood. And this arises likewise from the humors being cooked during the summer. And what remains from the cooking, when the heat is clearly extinguished, then becomes cold and dry; cold on account of the heat being extinguished, dry because of all the wetness being driven off during the cooking.

When winter takes over, the bile, being chilled, becomes less, and the phlegm increases again from the abundance of rain and from the length of the nights.

87-91. He means that in each of the four seasons, the prevailing humor is the one similar in mixture to that same season, and on this account names phlegm, cold and wet, as corresponding to winter, and blood, hot and wet, just like spring, and yellow bile, like summer he says to be hot and dry, and black bile, like autumn, to be cold and dry. It was shown earlier that he says each of the humors increases in its season, and now he gives the reason why phlegm is plentiful in the winter: "*from the abundance of rain,*" he says, "*and the length of the nights*", that is, on account of this season being so wet and cold. It is clear that it is wet from the abundance of rain, and cold from the length of the nights. The sun, approaching close to us at the highest point and making the day longer, is responsible for the heat of the air surrounding us, which prevails in the summer. In the same way, the sun is also responsible for the coldness of winter, when it is slanting, and lying low, and making its journey over the earth in a short time. Hippocrates assumes that the bodies of animals are affected by the composition of the air surrounding us, being dried out in dry mixtures of air, made wet in wet mixtures, and likewise heated in hot mixtures and chilled in cold mixtures. So, if winter is wet and cold, then phlegm, being wet and cold, logically increases then. And he has shown this earlier. And the account seems to agree with this for the other seasons, for yellow bile becomes plentiful in the summer, since it is fundamentally dry and hot, and in spring blood, which is the wet and hot humor, becomes plentiful (for he has said spring is also hot and wet) and in autumn black bile, being cold and dry like the season, becomes plentiful. Thus it is not an insignificant investigation which concerns the mixture of spring, how it is said to be hot and wet, which I have gone through in detail, showing that it is better to call it 'well-balanced'. And it is clear that blood, by this same reasoning, is not merely hot and wet, but well-balanced. Better yet would be an investigation which is omitted by commentators on this book, namely an investigation concerning phlegm being wet and cold in composition and also generated in winter. I will now tell you why I have said it is not an insignificant investigation. In the *Aphorisms* (1.15) Hippocrates himself says

the belly is by nature the hottest in the winter and spring, and sleep is the longest. And in this season food ought to be given plentifully. For there is plenty of innate heat and plentiful nourishment is needed. Those in the prime of life, and athletes, are evidence of this.
And again,
in the summer and autumn, foods are the most difficult to digest, in the winter the easiest, and in the spring the second easiest.

If this is true, and we know that phlegm is a cold humor, and not well-balanced like blood, how does it become plentiful in winter? For it is necessarily the case that blood, not phlegm, is generated from well-digested food. What is the solution to this difficulty? To me it seems to be this: the belly is hottest in winter with a heat by nature, that is, it is the best balanced, but parts of the body are more cold in winter: in some the stomach itself is cold due to a journey, or a lack of clothing, or particular pursuits or some such thing. At any rate, all the coldness of what is surrounding sinks for the most part, but in some it sinks to the location of the stomach, as has been said, so that, even if the food taken into the belly is well-digested during the change in the liver, it still does not take the precise form of blood-ness, but it fails somehow in making this change. Furthermore, the blood vessels in the entire body, when they have been chilled, similarly do not make this change. And the abundance of meat, which is served in the winter, enters in this way, along with the more phlegm-ish qualities. For people eat a great deal of pulse in the winter, and much more bread than in the other seasons, and wheat flour and honey cakes and thin cakes, and many turnips and meats – some clearly phlegm-ish, like mutton, and some only if not well-prepared, like pork and especially suckling pig. And through the entire winter people also eat vegetable bulbs and shellfish and eggs and cheese and many other phlegm-ish foods like these. And most people also drink new wine which is suitable to the creation of phlegm, so that phlegm increases for these reasons in the winter.

91.

The body of man contains all these things eternally, but from the revolving year now each of them becomes greater, and now lesser, depending on the part and on its nature.

91-92. The body of man, he says, possesses all these afore-said things, that is, the four humors, throughout its entire life. For this is what 'eternally' means in this context. But these humors become greater and lesser depending on the changes of the seasons. For this phrase "*from the revolving year*" signifies "changing", that is, "altering" and "settling" into some other season contained in the year. He says these things become "*greater*" and "*lesser*", "*depending on the part and on its nature.*" Some people, indeed, read the "*depending on the part*" as referring to all the parts of the body, and some read it in opposition to "*depending on its nature*", in which case the account would be as follows: the body of man always possesses the four previously mentioned humors, which are greater or lesser depending on the part of the year and its nature. And if someone were to say this with the order changed, he would have a useful thought, and true, besides. For most of the humors are exchanged according to the seasons, according to the nature of the corresponding season, and according to the part of the whole year. And if it is not managed according to nature, then a difference in the amounts of the humors arises. So it is allowable to read "*parts*" with respect to the year.

92.

For just as each year has a share in all the elements, so does the body – in the hot, the cold, the dry and the wet; none of these would last for any time at all without all the things existing in the universe. But if one were to fail, all would disappear, for they are all constructed due to the same necessity, and nourished from each other.

93-95. Hot and cold and dry and wet are not named or conceived of based on predominance, but he makes it clear in this passage when he calls them element-like and says that the entire year has a share in them all. For the entire year does not have a share in them all based on predominance, but has a share in them as element-like things: winter is entirely of wet and cold, and summer of the opposite, of dry and hot, and each of the other two seasons in opposition to each other, the one wet and hot, and the other cold and dry. And he shows this still more clearly by saying that if one of them were to be first to perish, the others would also be utterly destroyed. For it is true to say that, if one of the elements were to perish, then, with that one destroyed, the rest of them would also perish – but this is not true for elements based on predominance. In fact, the opposite is true: when something defined by predominance is destroyed, the opposite is preserved. For when it is summer, there is no winter; when winter, no summer; and when it is spring, no autumn; and when autumn, no spring. But if the hot element were absolutely destroyed, liquid would become solid, because heat would no longer exist, and the sun would perish completely, and nothing, neither plant not animal, would be left. Following this same reasoning, if the cold element were destroyed, everything would be fire; if the dry element were destroyed, everything would be water, and thus all the bodies generated in the universe would be destroyed. For this reason he says the element-like bodies are nourished from each other in this way. For the extreme element is thought of, rather than actually existing; but a certain one of the existing elements is almost the same. Indeed, if you were to imagine that wetness and cold in the extreme make water, then water would not yet be observed. For it would immediately solidify and stand still and cease flowing. And if you were to imagine earth as dryness and cold in the extreme, such a body would be harder than a diamond. And indeed, if earth were to become such, the generation of plants would cease, and with this generation ceasing, the nourishment of animals would be utterly lost, and if this happened it is clear that the animals themselves would perish. However, when the dry and cold elements are considered based on predominance, the earth in the universe is said to be a dry and cold body, and water is said to be a cold and wet body. And even fire itself also has a share in some air-like substance, just as also in some smoke-like substance, and yet it clearly requires liquid as nourishment, as the flames in lamps illustrate. For it is clear that the elements of the universe exist possessing nourishment from each other and for this reason, Plato says (*Timaeus* 33c7)

this one arises by design, having nourishment for itself from its own destruction, suffering and doing all things in itself and from itself.
95.
Thus, if one of these things born into man were to fail, the man would not be able to live.

95-97. He calls blood and phlegm and the biles inborn things, since the fetus takes its first composition from the blood of the mother, which has a share in all the humors, and it takes its growth and nourishment likewise. And if the wet element were entirely lost from our bodies, or the dry, or the hot, or the cold, the humors would immediately be destroyed according to the principle of domination, since they are not purely or extremely wet or dry or hot or cold. Indeed, we do not say that phlegm is wet and cold in that it has no share in the opposites (hot and dry), but in that it is dominated by wet and cold. If it were the extreme of cold only, it would be solidified like crystal, just as, if it were the extreme of wetness, it would have no thickness or viscosity. And it is the same way with the biles, for the yellow is said to be dry and fire-like, and the black to be dry and earth-like, yet clearly possessing wetness or it would not be a humor, but a solid body like diamond. Thus it is said to be cold in that there is more coldness in it than heat. For if it were the extreme of cold, it would be solidified in the manner of a crystal. And what needs to be said about the humors? For blood itself is said to seem to be the most well-balanced, because in it nothing dominates greatly over the other opposing humors, neither hot dominated by cold nor cold by hot, neither wet by dry, nor dry by wet. Blood itself, therefore, requires the four qualities (wetness, dryness, heat, and cold), and it is very clear that this will require a mixture of the other humors. And for this reason the most well-balanced blood is somewhat mixed with phlegm and yellow bile and black. And there is a certain physical theory, possessing no small persuasiveness, according to which the four humors are shown to be instrumental in the origin of characters suited to them. And it is necessary for it to be explained again that in this account the characters of the soul follow on the mixtures in the body, concerning which we have written elsewhere. This being assumed, therefore the sharp and intelligent character in the soul will be due to the bile-ish humor, the steadfast and firm character due to the melancholic humor, and the simple and stupid character due to blood. The nature of phlegm is most useless in the formation of character, and it appears to have its necessary origin in the first break-down of foods.

98.
In the year, sometimes winter prevails, then spring, then summer, then autumn. So also in man sometimes phlegm prevails, then blood, then bile, first the yellow, then the black.

This is clearly a passage written by a man trying to show that, just as in the year sometimes wetness and cold prevail, and such a season is called winter, then wetness and heat, when it is spring, then dryness and heat, which is named summer, and last after them the dry and cold in autumn – so also in man phlegm, the cold wet humor, dominates in the winter, and blood, the hot wet humor, in the spring, and yellow bile, dry and hot in its force, in the summer and in autumn black bile, dry and cold like autumn itself.

99.
The clearest proof is if you wish to give to the same man the same medicine four times in a year – he will vomit for you the most phlegm-ish matter in the winter, the most liquid in the spring, the most bile-ish in the summer and the blackest in the autumn.

He says that the "*clearest proof*" of the previous claim, according to which a given humor seems to prevail in each season of the year, is that when an emetic medicine is given to the same man four times, the vomited matter is most phlegm-ish in the winter, most liquid in the spring, most bile-ish in the summer and blackest in the autumn.

99-100.

And indeed it is necessarily so that these things are thus; that whatever diseases increase in winter become weaker in summer, and those that increase in summer, abate in winter – as long as they are diseases which are not recovered from in a matter of days alone. I will speak in turn about the period of days. And those diseases which arise in spring – it must be admitted that there is a recovery from them in autumn, and the diseases which arise in autumn, are necessarily recovered from in spring. When a disease goes beyond these seasons, one must realize that it will continue for a year.

100. The beginning of this passage possesses an ambiguous reading: some people reading "*opheilei...*" and some reading "*philei (goun touton houtos ekhonton)*" with the meaning "belong to, concern" For this word (i.e. *philei*) is sometimes used in place of *prosekei* (belong to, concern).

100-101. The rest of the passage is clear. He would have it that whatever diseases last not for a period of days, but reach a crisis in months, are recovered from in the season opposite to the season in which they arose; that is, in seven months, and if these are not thus recovered from he says the disease is a year-long one. And the term 'year-long' clearly can mean a disease recovered from one year after it has arisen, but it can also be after a period of seven years, as he says diseases are recovered from after a period of seven months. And indeed he spoke this way in the *Aphorisms* (3.28):

Most ailments suffered by children reach a crisis in forty days, but some reach it in seven months, and some in seven years, and some endure until maturity (101). "And it is necessary for a physician to make a stand against diseases, since each of them is strong in the body in that season which is most like it by nature.
"

101-102. He has now explained clearly in this present passage the utility of all the preceding discussion concerning seasons of the year, because the account has the same application to time of life and dwelling place and pursuits and daily regimen. For it is necessary that the physician, through careful observation, should try to make these things out: which humor is overabundant, predominating either with respect to amount or with respect to its own force, and in which part of the body particularly. In this way he may best accomplish his treatment, as is shown in *The Therapeutic Method*.

Concerning the Method in the Book and How It Belongs Among the Legitimate Works of Hippocrates

102-103. Hippocrates, proposing to find the nature of our bodies in this book, has used this method for the search: first he has inquired whether the nature is simple or complex, and then, having found that it is complex, he has considered the substance of the simple components in it – what sort of substance it is, that is, what power does it possess to be affected by something and to act, and in this way, on reflection, he has kept in mind the seasons and times of life – how the elements which have been discovered are related to these things. He found that the prognosis of recovery from diseases, and the treatments, necessarily refer back to these observations. And in his investigation of the compound elements of our body, he has kept in mind the elements themselves which exist in reality. For we sometimes loosely call the simple components in each thing according to its structure, as well as its primary parts, the 'elements' of this thing, just as people who speak of the harmonic and rhythmic and geometric and arithmetic elements of speech and voice and demonstration. And thus Plato says there are a hundred elements in a cart, having written that it was said by Hesiod: "*a hundred planks of the cart.*"

103-104. For all these things called 'elements' in this way are not, strictly speaking, simple and primary in each thing, but only those things which are common to all that exists are actually primary, and are correctly called 'elements.' Hippocrates named them based on their qualities: hot, cold, wet, and dry – these are not between the extremes, but are the extremes themselves, clearly fire, earth, water and air. Plato sees fit to represent this method thus, as well as what is observed concerning the nature of the soul: that nothing can be understood of them in part, without rigorously understanding the nature of the entire thing. I will cite for you this very passage of Plato's, reading thus:

If Hippocrates, of the Asclepiadian school, is to be trusted, the body cannot be understood except by this method.

He is correct, my friend. Still, it is necessary for us to examine logical reasoning with respect to Hippocrates, to see if it agrees.

All right.

What, then, does Hippocrates say that 'to observe concerning nature' is, and what does true reason say? For is it not necessary that the nature of anything whatsoever be understood in this way? First whether it is simple or complex. Then, if it is simple, to examine its power: what it possesses making it tend to act, and what tends to undergo its action. And if it has a complex form, then to examine it with respect to each individual aspect, in the same way as the simple was examined with respect to one aspect: what does it do by nature and what is affected by it.

104-106. But, seeing that Plato has written thus, let someone explain these things to us: in which other book of Hippocrates, besides the *On the Nature of Man*, does one find this same approach? Or, if someone is not able to explain this, let him seek no more trustworthy witness that this book is legitimate, than Plato. Moreover, Plato was born quite close in time to the students of Hippocrates, and if this book were by one of them, he would have given the author's name. For before the kings of Alexandria and Pergamon became so ambitious to possess ancient books, authorship was never falsely attributed. However, after the ones who collected the writings of a given ancient author for these kings first received a reward for this, they immediately collected many works, which they falsely inscribed. But these kings lived after the death of Alexander, and Plato wrote this passage before Alexander the Great, when these men had not yet treated the inscriptions dishonestly, but when each book displayed its particular author in a clear statement. Plato thus agrees that one must investigate concerning the nature of the soul using the Hippocratic method, as Hippocrates did concerning the nature of the body, and he says it is impossible for this investigation to be done well, before the nature of the entire man is known. Some people are mistaken in this, such that they think this wonderful method is from some other person, and they do not hesitate to write that the one who first discovered such a great and lofty process would neglect to explain it. For how is it not a great and lofty thing to discover the elements of all generated and perishable bodies? How is it not much better proven with explanations? And can these matters be apprehended, not in three hundred entire lines, but in far fewer? For it is not likely that, in all his therapeutic and prognostic discoveries, Hippocrates would nowhere use the afore-mentioned explanation for the elements being explained.

106-107. But I have stated these things at length when I showed that the book was a legitimate work of Hippocrates. And indeed, one should not be so concerned about this aspect in the work, but one should rather pay rigorous attention concerning the truth of what has been written in it. We have done this in the *On the Elements According to Hippocrates* – which these people who saw it was in good repute among the educated, and were envious, made a cold argument against, by saying that it was not a book by Hippocrates. However, it is agreed that he has proposed these things, and has written about them all in their turn, always with close attention. But since, out of shamelessness, envious ones argue against what is agreed on and believed by everyone, for this reason I have written another commentary and treatise which holds thus: that Hippocrates appears to have the same teaching in his other writings as in the *On the Nature of Man*.

108-109. I have expounded on the book itself *On the Nature of Man* in the first part of this work. Now I will turn to those things which have been incorrectly attached to it, added while the book was being assembled. For the added work is a single short book, in which the regimen of healthy people is discussed, and it seems to be the writing of Polybus, the student of Hippocrates. In addition, between this and the *On the Nature of Man*, something else has been compiled, and appended by the one who first joined these two short books into the same one, i.e. the *On the Nature of Man* of Hippocrates himself and the *Regimen of Health* of Polybus. For at the time when the Attalid and Ptolemaic kings were vying with each other in the acquisition of books, a recklessness began to arise with respect to the attribution and preparation of books on the part of those who, for money, brought back to the kings the writings of well-known men. For since both of these books are short, the *On the Nature of Man* and the *Regimen of Health*, some person, considering each of them to be negligible on account of their shortness, placed them both together in the same book. And perhaps some other person, or perhaps the same person who first joined them, inserted some material between the two, which we will now discuss.

110.
One should know these things about diseases: whatever diseases result from fullness, are cured by draining; the diseases generated by draining, are cured by fullness; the ones arising from exertion, are cured by rest and the ones caused by excessive idleness, are cured by exertion. With the knowledge of all this, the physician must stand in opposition to the constitutions and diseases and forms and seasons and times of life, and should loosen those things which tighten, and make tight those things which are loosened. In this way the sickness may be halted, and this seems to me to be the cure.

110-111. Beside every line of this entire passage, Dioscorides made the mark called the 'dagger' (Aristarchus used such a mark for those line of the Poet which he suspected). Dioscorides made this mark, inferring that the present passage was by Hippocrates, the son of Thessalos. For the great Hippocrates had two sons: Thessalos and Drakon, each of whom had a son Hippocrates. These remarks apply to the entire passage. Still, it is appropriate for us to consider this material to some extent, dealing with each phrase separately.

111-113.
Whatever diseases are caused by fullness, are cured by draining.

Saying that the necessary cause of diseases is fullness or draining or any of the other afore-mentioned things is not the same thing as saying that something arises on account of fullness or any of the others. For it is true that some diseases arise through fullness or as a consequence of fullness (for to say one or the other makes no difference), but it is not true that fullness is the necessary cause of the disease. For the disease itself is a certain condition in the body of the creature, which fundamentally harms the function, as is shown in the work, *On the Difference of Diseases*. But fullness does not fundamentally harm function, as has also been shown a while back in the work *On Fullness*. Rather, fullness causes harm through some intermediate condition, which Erasistratus has proposed arises in one way, Asclepiades in another way, and those physicians called 'Pneumatics' in yet another way. We have written further, how diseases arise from each fullness. For 'fullness' has been defined in two ways: the first way with respect to its fundamental property, and the second with respect to the capacity of vessels. Fullness, as it is defined with respect to fundamental property, leads the humors into corruption and sends a stream into the weakest parts in the body. On the other hand, fullness defined by volume causes openings and ruptures of the vessels, and sometimes sudden death, whenever it blocks up the body's transpirations. The term 'healing' may be used in reference to those things causing the diseases, not only to those diseases which have already arisen. If, indeed, someone were to use the proper term with reference to them, he would say that such causes are preconditions of diseases, just as Athenaeus does. And again, these same preconditions, those which he calls 'previously-completed' and 'starting-before', arise in turn from the following: poor digestion of large amounts of meat, followed by visits to the public baths and gymnasium at unpropitious times, and by all the things which I discussed in the treatise *On the Previously-Completed Causes*: these become agents of the preconditioning causes of each disease.

113-114.
The diseases caused by draining, are cured by fullness.

The writer of this passage doesn't seem to have used the term 'fullness' correctly here, since not only all physicians, but all the other Greeks as well, are accustomed to assign the term 'fullness' to excesses of a well-balanced quantity, and emptiness is not rectified through a corresponding imbalance. Hear next the argument advocating opposing imbalances. Since certain foods are well-balanced depending on one's constitution, the lack or the abundance within a healthy person will be comprehended by a comparison to these foods. Whoever is emptied, if he is to be restored, will be increased by that amount of well-balanced material which was present there earlier. For if the same amount of food would be brought in now, as was being brought in before the draining, that which was drained would never be restored in full. But it is the mark of a skilled practitioner that the increase of this be made in a balanced way and that what was drained off not be filled at a crisis point, and not suddenly all at once. Some physicians teach that drainings are never the causes of diseases. They say that drainings only cause a weakening of strength, and a wasting away of the outside of the body, and that no disease arises from deficiency. But they haven't seen those diseases which arise from imbalanced drainings. When this happens, the patients readily become chilled, and quickly feverish again, and are easily overpowered by fatigue and all the external afflictions, so that even those who are healthy are led into illness by sleeplessness and distress and indigestion and temper.

114.
Whatever diseases arise from exertion are cured by rest.

What he calls 'exertions' are those exertions arising from ill-balanced motion. And indeed, that motions which treat the body in this way should be halted, is something which all men know, and they act accordingly, without being obliged to consult a physician. And we have shown, that not only men, but even irrational creatures rectify a harmful situation through methods opposite to it.

115.

Whatever diseases arise from excessive idleness are cured by exertion.

Idleness does not cause disease primarily and in itself, but by means of excess. For parts of the body characterized by idleness become weaker and less robust, as each excess comes about due to this idleness. Moreover, an ill-balanced motion does not make the power stronger, but it does empty out the excess liquids which have been collected. For it is quite clear that if there is a slight over-fullness with respect to this abundance of liquids, or a well-balanced motion takes place, a man becomes worn out gently through this, but does not become feverish.

115-116.

With the knowledge of all this, the physician must stand in opposition to the disease: the form and season and time of life...

He seems to say 'form' as equivalent to the nature of the body, the substance of which we have shown to consist of a mixture of four elements. Indeed it has been demonstrated that all diseases are cured by opposition to their fundamental properties, not to their immediate symptoms. And the nature of the body, since it is a mixture, is not entirely corrected through oppositions, just as the seasons and times of life are not. For some people are born well-balanced, as others are born ill-balanced, and the good balance of the former is preserved by similar things and the ill-balance of the latter corrected by opposing things. And these things are defined in the procedure, *On Healthy People.*

116-117.

...and loosen those things which tighten, and make tight those things which are loosened.

He hasn't made a proper comparison of the diseases here. For 'things which loosen' is normally considered a counterpart to 'things which tighten', and 'things which are tightened' to 'things which are loosened.' For 'things which tighten' and 'things which loosen' are properly said in reference to the causes of disease, not in reference to the bodies themselves which are being harmed. Contrariwise, 'things which are tightened' and 'things which are loosened' are said in reference to bodies already being harmed. So 'things which are tightened' and 'things which are loosened' are terms not for diseases, but for the bodies being tightened or loosened, just as are the terms 'hard', 'soft', 'thin', 'thick', concerning which the eighth book of the *Epidemics* speaks well in this passage:

...softening of hard skin, loosening of skin which is tightened...

117. For in this book, 'being compressed' is spoken of with reference to 'holding together', and is the opposite of 'being made thin', just as 'being thickened' is the opposite. For this, in turn, has the same force as 'being thickened', just as 'having been thickened' has the same force as 'having been compressed'.

117.

Some diseases arise from regimen, and some from the air which we inhale as we live.

People sometimes refer to food and drink alone as 'regimen', but most often they include activities in this term, and it will be considered as defined in this way here. For diseases arise not only from what we eat and drink, but also public baths and activities at the gymnasium, and sleeplessness, and distress, and anger, and chills, and overheating. And harm often arises "*from the air*" alone as it is inhaled, such as in those places called 'the regions of Charon'.

118.

The diagnosis of each disease should be made in this way: when many men are stricken by one disease at the same time, the cause should be assigned to that which is the most common and which we all make use of. And this is that which we breathe. For it is clear, that the regimens of each of us cannot be the cause since the disease has been contracted by everyone in turn, the young and the old, the men and the women, drinkers and non-drinkers, wheat-eaters and bread-eaters, those exerting themselves heavily and those exerting themselves little. So regimen cannot be the cause when men living in so many different ways are stricken with the same disease. But whenever diseases of all types arise at the same time, it is clear that the individual regimens are the cause of each disease.

118-119. He says correctly that diseases common to many have a common cause, just as he is correct about other things in this passage, but he is not correct in assigning the origin of all common diseases to air alone, if indeed,

Those in Ainos eating pulse during a famine became weak in the limbs, while those eating vetch-seeds suffered pains in the knees. (Epidemics 2.4.3.2, also 6.4.11.2)

And we know that some people, compelled by famine to eat half-rotten wheat, were stricken by a common disease from a common cause, and we know how an entire encampment using wretched water had a similar illness among all the soldiers. But the rest of the passage is clear.

119-121.

...and the treatment must be carried out in opposition to the cause of the disease, as I have said elsewhere, and there must be a change in regimen. For it is clear that the type of life the man is accustomed to lead is not suitable, either entirely or in most respects, or in some single respect. These things, once they have been discovered, should be changed, and the treatment should be performed based on the observation of the man's time of life and his body type, and the season of the year, and the kind of disease; sometimes removing, sometimes adding, as I have said before. And it is necessary to make alterations in the

medicine and regimen based on each of these: time of life, season of the year, body type and disease. But when the epidemic of a single disease prevails, it is clear that the regimen is not the cause, but rather that which we breathe, and it is clear that it possesses some noxious vapor. And at such a time, this advice should be given to men: not to change their regimen, which is not the cause of the disease, but to look to their body, that it may be as thin and as weak as possible, gradually reducing the food and drink which they are accustomed to consume. For if the regimen should be changed abruptly, there is a risk of some newer danger in the body from this change. But it is necessary that the regimen be followed in such a way that it is clear that there is nothing harming the man. And it is necessary to be mindful of the breath, that the airflow into the body be as slight as possible and as distant as possible, exchanging those places in which the disease prevails for ones of a different type, and reducing the body, for on that account men will need less plentiful breathing and less deep.

121-122. He has written that a cure for common diseases is lacking when they arise from the surroundings. For although certain vapors from marshes or swamps or wetlands often become causes of such diseases, still, sometimes it is the mixture of seasons alone. With reference to the vapors, he has written a therapy correctly, for the most specific quality of the entire matter, rather than for the single quality of those who are suffering bodily afflictions, and he has devised this therapy with two aims, a change of location and the practice of lighter inhalation. However, with reference to people who are stricken because of their quality, there should not only be a treatment of diseases which have already arisen, but also a prevention against them arising at all, by means of opposing qualities; if the body would be harmed by excessive heat, it can be prevented by cooling, if harmed by a chill then prevented by heating, and the same principle for the other qualities, both simple and compound. I have already spoken before concerning the indication of diseases by time of life and seasons and proportions of the body.

122. This "*...to make alterations in medicine...*" seems to me to have been written here in place of "to apply medicine" to the disease from an opposition. For currently in Asia a man is said to "be altered" in this way: usefully or kindly or suspiciously or harshly.

122-123.
Whatever diseases arise from the strongest parts of the body are the deadliest. For if the disease remains in the place where it began, it is necessarily the case that, as the strongest part suffers, the entire body is disturbed. And if the disease should come to one of the weaker parts from the stronger, it is difficult to expel. But whatever disease goes from the stronger to the weaker, is easily released. For the flux is easily locked out by the strength.

123-128. If someone wished to say either a part or a body was 'strongest', he would properly name that one best equipped for strenuous action, the same way that we say that Hercules was born the strongest. But in another way we say that one body or one part is strong with respect to one activity, and another body or part with respect to another activity. For although in general there is strength in the body for each activity, nevertheless for any given activity, one part as opposed to another becomes the strongest. For this is one activity: the movement of a living thing by impulse, such as the movement of something running, or struggling with some living creature, or pulling apart some body, living or dead, or dragging in some way. And there is one other power, and vital activity with respect to this power, according to which the arteries and the heart pulse. With respect to those activities differing from each other in type, some others are distinct, not only in animals, but even in plants, so we call them natural forces: drawing, altering, holding and separating. So, for example, sometimes it happens that the stomach may have the strongest power in one body or another with respect to the activity of either holding or of altering, and then at some time the liver or spleen or one of the others is strongest. Contrariwise, the stomach may have the weakest power in this same body with respect to drawing and separating, and the liver may have the strongest. And the person who wrote this passage concedes that a part seems to be strong in us, to the extent that it does not easily suffer from disease-generating causes.

Further, by God, this is added, i.e. a part is strong to the extent that, when some abundance of humors has collected in it, it is able to send this abundance into another part, by means of the separating power. For clearly the sender must be stronger than the receiver. Let there be, for example, some weakest part for each body, and some strongest part, as is certainly agreed on by all physicians and laymen. For they say that the feet are weakest for those with gouty feet, just as the joints are for arthritics, and the head for headache sufferers; just as the spleen is for those splenetic by nature and the eyes for those affected with eye-diseases, and so on for each part. Given that the disease-producing causes are of two kinds (the one external, the other driven by our own selves); with respect to ailments from the outside, some parts of our body are sometimes weak, and with respect to diseases from the inside, other parts are weak, since the powers of the causes themselves are of different kinds. For diseases arise internally through an abundance or wretchedness of humors, while some external causes harm the bodies of living things through making an ill-balance, and others harm by bruising or cutting. To be sure, the suffering of those with dislocations seems to arise from both. For one man, by himself without touching another, suffers a dislocation either by going to his knees or opening his jaws or somehow either exerting or twisting one of the other joints. And before now someone has suffered a fracture without any external causes, from contorted twistings or excessive leaps. For as many as are the kinds of causes, there are just as many kinds of weakness and strength in the parts of the body which suffer easily, or which do not suffer. For the diseases impelled by the humors all arise according to the strength and weakness of the separating powers. So, among similar parts of a creature, the disease-working humors go from the ones most able to reject them into others, and then from those into others, until they settle in some one of the weakest, which has no part weaker than it anywhere into which it might send the offending humor. And if this part has some exit-passage, as the intestines and stomach and bladder and uterus do, the offending cause is poured out through excretion. And if it should be lighter in composition than the passages of that part, then often the draining comes about with the vessel having been greatly torn or opened, as among those bleeding profusely without any trauma. If it is not opened or torn, the heavy, viscous humor descends and makes a mass in the part according to its nature. In this way, there is a certain strength and weakness of the parts of the body for those sufferings which have originated in ourselves. But the parts suffering from external causes seem to suffer generally with respect to being heated and chilled and dried and made wet. For those things leading the bodies of living things into disease by means of bruising or cutting or doing some such thing are rare. Moreover, one is born weak and strong with respect to one and another of these such diseases. For whatever parts are colder by nature, these are affected easily by chilling causes; the hotter ones, by heating; and the some logic applies to those imbalances with respect to wetness and dryness. For it is demonstrated that although some parts suffer readily from heating or chilling or drying or wetting causes, nevertheless there is another stronger part able to efficiently send off its own suffering into these weaker ones.

128. Since 'stronger' part and 'weaker' part are not spoken and thought of simply, but in many different ways, it is not possible to evaluate this passage nor to know whether it is true or false. But it is possible to say one thing with reference to this passage, and with reference to all the others written about things which are often said and thought ambiguously: that their account is so confused and inarticulate, that no one in the audience is helped by it.

128-130. And indeed there is a strong counter-argument against this passage, where he says

whichever diseases go from the weaker to the stronger are the most easily released. For the flux is easily locked out by the strength.

Wherefore, exegetes have written different explanations of *apokleizetai* (is locked out): some taking it as *apokleizetai*, some as *apokleietai* (is shut out), and some as *apopagiosetai* (is curdled), expanding the third syllable from the end of the verb *apopagiosetai* with the omega, some with eta and sigma, just as Dioscorides says this verb is taken from *pagesesthai* (to be made solid), instead of *apokrouesthai* (to be beaten away). But the offending humor, driven from the weakest parts to one of the strongest parts, would be repelled in turn and nothing much would happen from this to someone suffering thus. It is better to write the passage in this way: "for the flux is released by the strength,' that is, having been cooked and altered, it is released. Some, making a false argument, say that the most essential parts are the strongest. For it is best for the offending humors to be moved from the most essential parts to the less essential, not from the less essential to the more. For we often observe, that when humors are carried into the limits and repelled into the joints and feet, if they go into some essential part there is only one hope of saving the dying man, and that is if we should be able to drive the humors back into the limb.

130-132.

The thickest blood vessels are arranged in this way: there are four pairs in the body, and the first of them reaches from the back of the head through the outside of the neck and along the inside of the spine and inside to the loins, and into the upper legs, and then it passes through the lower legs to the ankles on the outside and into the feet. Bloodlettings to treat pains in the back and loins should be made from the hams and the outside of the ankles. The second pair of vessels, having its origin from the head by the ears, through the neck, is called the jugular: they go from the inside of the belly along the spine on either side, and along the loins and into the testicles and into the thighs, and through the hams from the inner part, and then through the lower legs to the inner ankle and into the feet. Bloodlettings against pains in the loins and testicles should be made from the hams and the inner ankles. The third pair goes from the temples through the neck under the shoulder blades; then they are carried to the lungs and one reaches from the right to the left and the other from the left to the right. And the right-hand one goes from the lungs below the breast and into the spleen and the kidney, while the one from the left goes into the right-hand side through the lungs below the breast and into the liver and the kidney, and they both end in the anus. The fourth pair goes from the front of the head and eyes under the neck and collar bones, and then from the upper side of the upper arms into the elbows and then through the fore-arms into the wrists and fingers, then from the fingers back through the hands and upper side of the fore-arms into the elbows and through the lower side of the upper arms into the armpits and from the upper ribs one reaches the spleen and the other reaches the liver, and then they both end by going over the stomach into the genitals. And this is how the major vessels are. And there are also vessels from the belly, of many sorts and in many places all over the body, through which nourishment comes to the body.

132-134. Of matters in dispute based on skill, observation decides some, and reasoning decides others. Things decided by observation, therefore, require a finely discerning observation, and those decided by reasoning require a well-trained argumentation. Concerning the digestion of foods in the stomach, and after that, the generation of humors and the distribution and nourishing, and with respect to other such things, we lack an argumentation to determine the opinions written by the ancients. To know whether ruminants have four stomachs and sheep have one, observation is required, not reasoning. On the other hand, both matters decided by observation and those decided by reason possess a way of testing what is untrue. For although matters decided by observation bring the readiest decision to those disagreeing with each other, based on the evidence from dissections, nevertheless those decided by reasoning can be decided from written arguments without dissection. So, if someone is compelled to use written works to argue against people who boldly assert the most shameless and uneducated things concerning some anatomical theory which should be decided by observation, those who are not familiar with the evidence from dissection are unable to distinguish what is false from what is true. For, just as if someone were to say that Crete is not an island, he would be scorned by all of those listening, since they would know it is an island, so too if someone were to say that dogs have four stomachs, but ruminants have one, he would be laughed at in the presence of those who have seen the four stomachs in ruminants and the single one in dogs. And it is the same thing with the dissection of blood vessels. For the decision requires observation, not reasoning. And until those who differ in opinion from the passage above write their own works, just as they wish, the truth will continue to be unclear to those who have not performed dissection.

134-138. We, who have reached such a different opinion from those who dare to say in this present account that four pairs of vessels reach from the head into the body, are unable to give a strong argument from written sources to those people who are ignorant of matters with respect to dissection, because this decision requires knowledge from observation alone, not from logical reasoning entirely – we are unable to give a strong argument, that is, unless someone selects those writings concerning the investigation of judgment by other physicians and philosophers (not the least of whom are the Empiricists), and is willing for the judgment to be made according to these writings he has selected. For I do not avoid other such tests and consensus of investigators, especially if they are experienced in the matter being investigated, such as Eudemus, and Herophilus the dissector, and Crateuas and Dioscorides of pharmaceutical metals. For if someone shuns this sort of judging, not only will they be unable to demonstrate that there are eight vessels coming from the head, but not even that there are three or two. For there is a single greatest vessel, which they call *koilic*, stretched through the lobes of the liver along the length of the living creature, clearly passing through the diaphragm region of the creature below and above. This same *koilic* vessel is carried up through the diaphragm region to the heart, and also down to the spine, entering in against the lobe of the liver, and then all of the vessels of the upper diaphragm are clearly seen springing from the vessel carried up as if from a tree trunk, while those of the lower diaphragm spring from the vessel curved against the spine. These things have even been written by Hippocrates in the second book of the *Epidemics*: he called the *koilic* vessel the *hepatic* and it is written in this way by all the anatomists. For no other physician says there are eight vessels leading from the head down into the body, not among those performing dissections less carefully and not among those performing them very carefully, neither Diocles, nor Praxogoras, nor Erasistratus, nor Pleistonicus, nor Philotimus, nor Mnesitheus, nor Dieuches, nor Chrysippus, nor Aristogenes, nor Medeius, nor Euryphon nor any other of the ancient physicians. And what is there yet to say concerning those who have added to the anatomical theory after them, like Herophilus and Eudemus, to whom no one has yet added anything in methodology, up to Marinus and Nomisianus, not even Heracleianus, who was my contemporary, but not my colleague, in Alexandria. For there are many students of these men, and others, the most distinguished being my teacher Pelops (student of Nomisianus), and Quintus, student of Marinus. But although Quintus wrote no book on anatomy or anything else, nevertheless we do have not a few books of anatomy by all the others. And there are anatomical writings by the students of Quintus, such as Satyrus, and our teacher, and Lykus. So, of all of these, and of the many anatomical writers besides them, no one recognizes four pairs of vessels leading from the head. For this is like saying there are eight Acropolis' in the city of Athens when there is only one. Indeed, it is possible for someone to say that there are eight inhabited hills in Rome, just as someone may say there are six. For each of them is off by one. But if someone were to say that there is one inhabited hill, instead of seven, or on the other hand, that there are eight Acropolis' in Athens instead of one, they would differ from someone telling the truth by much more than one. Thus, since there is one single vessel carried up from the lobes of the liver into the upper body (or if someone starts the dissection from above, it is said to be carried down rather than carried up, but still one single vessel is observed), someone saying that eight vessels are carried down from above would be most ridiculous. For whether you wish to say that the *hepatic* or the *koilic* vessel is carried below from above, or carried above from below, it is still the same single one stretched through the lobes of the liver. So if some anatomy book by someone else has been found having such an opinion, no one has taken the opinion further, nor dared to acknowledge it step by step. Rather, upon hearing this one proposal, that there are four pairs of vessel in the body, anyone would condemn it as if stunned, and immediately withdraw from the proposition. But since someone has added this writing to the treatise of Hippocrates, we have been forced to allow this much time to be lost, as we are still spending arguing against this opinion, and have spent before now, inasmuch as we recognize that these things are wretchedly written.

138-142. He says that a pair of blood vessels starts from the back of the head, and is carried through the neck, and then, traveling from the outer parts along the spine to the loins, from there goes through the leg into the outside of the ankle. And he says that another, second pair arises from the places near the ear, and goes through the throat, being known as the jugular veins, and then, like the first pair, from the outer parts along the spine, so it then goes from there inside to the testicles and thighs, and then reaches through the knees and to the ankles on the inside. Who, having seen the dissection of animals, on hearing these things would admit them for even one day? For although there are many poorly explained observations in dissections, concerning which it is reasonable that someone might make a mistake since they have not completely thrashed it out in practice, and for this reason disagreements concerning them have arisen, still the sight of the greatest blood vessel is so clear, that no one who has been able to learn anything from dissection would be able to overlook it. This is agreed on by everyone to such an extent that even the poets know it. Indeed, Homer says:

He cut away that entire blood vessel which, placed at the top of the back, reaches entirely through the neck (Iliad 13.546-547).

Therefore he knew there is one single vessel, as in fact there is, not four vessels with two from the outside of the spine, and two more at the same spot stretching alongside them on either side of the spine. But no creature possesses four vessels as the fabricator of the anatomy described here has written. Instead, the blood supply for whatever is between the limits of the back comes from the single great blood vessel, as Hippocrates wrote in the second book of the *Epidemics*:

The upper limit of it against the collarbones, and the lower limit against the eighth vertebra

and the upper splits into the jugular veins, and the lower into the vessels carried into the legs. For how could the one who wrote about this second pair suppose that the two jugular veins, persevering, are carried along the spine out from the inner parts to the legs? How could they reach the ankles? For, since there is one single large vessel leading into each of the legs, it is not the case that the vessels of the inside of the ankles come from one vessel, and those of the outside of the ankle from another; but rather they are all offshoots of this very vessel. Even more laughable than these is the third pair, which he says originates in the temples and is carried through the neck beyond the shoulder-blades into the lungs and then from there the two members of the pair exchange the straightforwardness of their direction, and are turned to the side, the one from the right-hand parts going to the left, and then reaching below the breast to the spleen and the left kidney, while the one from the left-hand parts goes to the right, then under the breast to the liver and right kidney. And both end in the anus. But the anus, my brilliant friend, as someone arguing against the writer of these things would be likely to say, receives a bloodstream from the entrails in this spot at the loins, whence it happens that the bloodstreams of the belly in each part are carried into the legs like some great conduits. Moreover, what physician, what butcher even, is unaware that blood is carried from the heart to the lungs through a single vessel. But the inventor of this third pair makes no mention of the heart anywhere in his account. Rather the present treatise assumes that the heart, which some dissectors say is the source of all the blood vessels in the body, possesses not one blood vessel. For he has said that the fourth pair originates from the front of the head and the eyes, and goes past the neck pressed against the collar bones, to the arms, namely to each individual hand, and then from the upper parts becomes entangled in the fingers, and is carried back through the entire hand and arm to the armpit, and from there goes through the ribs, one to the liver, the other to the spleen, and then, carried from the stomach, they both end in the genitals, so that they give no share whatever to the heart. How, finally, could the one fabricating these things like a young Prometheus have overlooked such an important organ as the heart? Indeed, he made no mention of the brains. For clearly this is less noble than the ankles! And beyond all this even is the blindness with respect to the kidneys, to which great vessels are carried from the belly; overlooking these, he has imagined that some vessels are carried from the lungs to the kidneys. So it is clear from all these things that he has not merely mis-observed, as some dissectors have mis-observed some things, but that he has observed nothing at all. For someone who does not observe the most important things is truly not described as mis-observing, but as not observing at all.

142-144. No one who has set to work at all observing something at dissections would be unaware that his theory about vessels being carried down from the head into the whole body is like a drunken hallucination. For although it is likely that dissectors may mis-observe some small blood vessels, someone would certainly not write another, entirely different account, nor leave out things which can be distinguished by blind men, as it were, using their fingers to touch. In truth, there is one vessel, through which blood is carried from the liver into the entire body, with small vessels branching off from the liver like many shoots from a trunk, which carry the blood to all the parts of the creature. And if you compare the blood in the belly to a river, and compare that which is carried from it into the parts of the body to a pipe, you will not be mistaken in this image. But if someone were to say that the large blood vessel is like a river or tree trunk, every physician would agree that this is a single vessel, except for the one who has audaciously added four pairs of vessels in this book. For in contrast to the others, just as he has allowed the heart to be overlooked, so also he ignores the *koilic* vessel, although he does remember the jugulars, into which it is split at the upper neck. For the large vessel dominates whatever is between this place and the limits of the spine, having offshooting vessels on either side. It is split in two at each of the limits of its parts: at the top, large vessels are carried through the throat, called jugular, and at the bottom, as has been said, one single large vessel is carried to each leg. But when he made note of the vessels carried through the throat, the jugulars, in the second pair, this young Prometheus showed great ignorance and boldness by nowhere noting the *koilic* vessel as it splits, from which these jugulars arise. For if he had seen the smallest thing in dissections, he would have had to say that the jugulars, going towards each other, end in this one vessel, the *hepatic* vessel, or *koilic* vessel, or whatever else someone may want to call it. But the argument was written by someone saying that two vessels. perservering, are carried through the inner parts along the spine to the insides of the ankles.

144-146. Why, then, would anyone make note of the vessels which he has written about after the four pairs? He claims that these carry nourishment from the belly into the entire body, as if the afore-mentioned four pairs were generated for some other function by nature, and did not have the single function common to all blood vessels: to carry blood from the liver to all the parts of the creature. For not one of those distributing the juices from food, from the belly and intestines into the liver, goes further than the liver. But they do not seem to be at many places in the liver, although they are great in number, attending to the stomach and other intestinal organs. Rather, they all reach to one spot, which is called the 'portals' of the liver: the one who first assigned the term 'portals' to this place was comparing the liver to a city or to some great dwelling, and the intestinal organs to the fields from which the food is carried into the gates of the city or dwelling as if through many roads, the blood vessels. But the young Prometheus is foolish in this creature which he has concocted according to his own theory. For someone would not make up a creature with these attributes, a creature in which the vessels carry nourishment from the intestinal organs directly into the body. For in fact they all reach into one spot, the portals of the liver, and from there the vessels receive the nourishment prepared in this organ, and go out again to the *koilic* vessel from which, as I said a little above, the blood is distributed into the entire body

146.
They also carry from the thick vessels into the belly and into the rest of the body from the outside and from the inside, and they give to each other; from the inside to the outside and from the outside to the inside.

146-148. Four pairs of vessels are enough for the young Prometheus, but he is not satisfied, and from greediness he has disgraced himself by adding to these the vessels carrying nourishment from the belly into the body. Now he has added to the argument a colophon about the common features of blood vessels, saying nothing true. For not one of these vessels flowing from the koilic vessel, which he terms 'thick', seems to be distributed into another pair flowing in the belly or internal parts. But just as the fabricator of these things had said nothing true in the anatomy which he proposed, neither entirely, nor in even one passage, so Hippocrates says nothing untrue at all in the second book of the *Epidemics*. But those who attempt to make an exegesis of the books of Hippocrates, not grasping even the outline of anatomy, are out of their minds, and especially those calling themselves Hipppocratics, who suppose that all this nonsense on the anatomy of blood vessels, and the second book of the *Epidemics*, were both written by the same man. If indeed something additional were to be theorized concerning the second of these, it is possible that the same man, with the passage of time, becoming more skilled with respect to what he had written first, would judiciously set out a second work. But then Hippocrates himself would seem to have described meticulously not only those things clearly visible to all, but also to have mis-observed things which even someone performing a dissection without sight should discover by touch – how is it possible for the same man to have written both of these? By what logic would someone, having written an argument concerning the elements of man, tack on to it in turn a discussion about blood vessels? For either one should write about anatomy in its entirety, or not write about blood vessels. Although such a variety of theory is acceptable in outlines which we write for our own recollection, nevertheless in a treatise it is not at all acceptable for some part of a second teaching to be added to the first after it has been completed, and then, a little later, to write the remainder about something a bit different, or entirely different, as is the case with these things attached to the book *On the Nature of Man*.

148.

Bloodlettings should be performed according to these principles.

149. He has already said these things clearly about the first pair of vessels, having set this down at the end in this sentence:

Bloodlettings for pains in the back and loins should be made from the hams and from the outside of the ankles,

and adding this to the second pair of vessels:

Bloodlettings for pain in the genitals and testicles should be made from the hams and the inside of the ankles.

He does not say anything about bloodletting with reference to the third and fourth pairs, in the same way as he constructed a defective account about these things, omitting many parts of the body in which he ought to have said there are vessels to be opened. But just as he has written detaching some small piece of the entire subject of anatomy, so also he detached the accounts concerning bloodletting.

149-150.

One must be careful to make the cuttings of the vessels as far as possible from the places where the pains have been discovered to originate, and the blood to collect. In this way the change will be the least far-reaching and sudden, and you will change the habitual course, so that the blood will no longer collect in the same spot.

150. The exegetes have understood correctly, that he says 'cuttings' in reference to what we describe with the compound word 'bloodlettings'. And they all agree on this: that he has not further differentiated whether he approves of opposition to flowing humors starting when the parts of the body are already in pain, or starting in a period of health. And for this someone might blame him. But it seems to me that he is speaking about healthy people, and assuming that the excessive humors are carried into other parts.

150-152.

The ones who spit up a great deal of pus without there being a fever, and the ones who have a great deal of pus standing in their urine, without pain, and the ones with bloody evacuations, just as among those with dysentery, with this persisting for a long time, and they being thirty-five or older – to all of these a spontaneous disease has arisen. For it must be the case that they were hardworking, exerting their body, and diligent when they were young, and then later, removed from their toils, they became fleshy with a soft flesh very different from before, and their body is quite changed, from the earlier one to the one which it has become, so that there is no correspondence. So, when some disease strikes men in this condition, they escape to begin with, but later, after the disease, their body wastes away in time, and ichor-like material flows through the vessels where they happen to be the broadest. If it presses on to the lower belly, then the fecal matter becomes like the matter which is inside the body, for since the path goes down, this material does not stand long in the bowel. For those into whose chest it flows, suppuration arises. For since the exit is going upwards, it sits for a long time in the chest and becomes pus-like. For those in whom it empties into the bladder, it becomes white due to the heat of that place, and separates, and the lightest goes up and the heaviest goes down and is called 'pus'.

152-153. All the things said in this passage are clear and should be paid attention to, without an exegete interpreting. And if they are all true, they should be put to the test of observation and the test of logic. As for the test of observation: it is to see if some people without fever are observed either coughing up pus or excreting something in their urine, and in addition to this, if they were hardworking in their earlier life, but now have ceased working for some time, and if when they were sick they survived, but later these afore-mentioned pus-like excretions afflicted them. By logic, it can be decided whether the cause from which the writer says these things have occurred is true or false. It is clear to those experienced in the explanatory method that the things said by this author are not so by necessity. For if this account had a persuasiveness, then each person would see it for himself. Concerning the observations of experience, I may say this to you that I have seen bloody excretions from the stomach occur not infrequently in those who have put an end to the habit of strenuous exercise, but never pus-like excretions. I have often seen mucus-like excretions from the stomachs of these men, in both wasted and healthy periods, as also the material coughed up has been putrefied, but it is not pus-like.

153.

Stones occur in children because of the heat of that place and of the entire body.

154. "*Of that place*", clearly meaning "of the bladder", concerning which he wrote thus at the end of the first passage: "*For those into whose bladder it flows, it becomes white due to the heat of that place.*" So he says that stones occur in children because of the heat of the bladder and of the entire body, and then he speaks next about the heat of children.

For one must know well, that man is hottest on his own account at the beginning of his life, and coldest at the end.

154-155. The account of those who say simply without qualification that man is hottest at the beginning of his life is not true, but with a qualification it is true. For he is hottest, if it is derived from an 'innate quality'. And this is the case with most children. The writer of this present passage has misunderstood the most crucial thing in this account, as will be clear from the following passage. For he has not realized, as Hippocrates said, that "*those things growing the most possess a hot innate quality*", and Hippocrates himself understands it so, but without this term "*innate quality*", he would have simply thought that growing things were hot.

155.

For it is necessarily the case that the body which is growing and spreading is hot due to the life-force.

155-156. Although Hippocrates says "*those things growing most possess a hot innate quality*", this person seems to have understood simply that for things which are growing the body is hot, without the term "*innate quality*" being added to the account. For he says that this very 'spreading' comes about due to the "*hot life-force*". And he wants to explain such a spreading due to life-force in this way: it seems to him that growth is some vigorous and vital action, and further, that just as other vigorous actions heat the one performing them, so growth does as well. But, on the contrary, he should have said that children grow due to the hot innate quality, not that they become hot due to the growth. For the hot innate quality is not only well-balanced with respect to heat, but also with respect to wetness. Thus such bodies, grown naturally for things which are extending in three dimensions, as if dispersing, take the increase in all these dimensions. Nature, therefore, extends these dimensions in every organ innately suited for this, using the heat. For it is readily extended by means of wetness. Indeed, many children, when they eat large amounts, concentrate the humor specifically termed 'raw', from which stones easily arise, since, although this humor from which the stone is formed possesses a name taken from its material, nevertheless, the productive cause is from heat.

156. *"But when the body begins to waste away, running down easily, it becomes colder."*

156-157. Here again, when the body no longer grows for those past their prime, he says that it becomes colder due to idleness. But, on the contrary, there is a better explanation of the cause. For as the hot innate quality becomes less in the body, the growth ceases. The author of these things has made his own opinion clearer in the following passage:

157.
And according to this account, inasmuch as a man grows the most at the beginning of his life, so he becomes hottest then, and at the end of his life, inasmuch as he wastes away, so he necessarily is coldest.

We have correctly explained the passage in which he said

...for it is necessarily the case that a body which is growing and spreading is hot due to the life-force.

For, on the contrary, he ought to have said that the growing thing grows due to the hot innate quality, not that it becomes hot due to growth. It is analogous to this for someone past their prime, when they are no longer growing: he thinks that the coldness arises due to a resting from the earlier action of growth which has now ceased.

158.
People in this condition become healthy spontaneously; most of them doing so in a space of forty-five days after they began to ail, but whichever ones exceed this period of time, will spontaneously become healthy in one year, if the patient is not attacked in some other way.

158-160. Who are the ones he says are *"in this condition"*? He clearly refers to those who, having stopped exercising due to idleness, cough up and urinate pus, and are afflicted with dysentery. Although I have said that I have seen many who have exchanged their earlier life of exertion and toil for a sedentary one, afflicted with bloody dysentery, yet I have not seen any of these coughing up or urinating pus. But he seems to me to be saying that the humor termed 'raw', when it has undergone coction, is pus. Why is this to be marveled at, when even Erasistrates supposes that the sediments in urine are not this humor, but pus, not knowing that such matter often settles out for the heavy eaters among healthy people. Indeed, over the course of time, we have seen a variety of matter resembling that which is called mucus excreted in the urine, in various kinds of men leading idle lives. And for some of these people, the excreted matter, having made a slow passage, seems to resemble pus, just as for those who bring up pus when they breathe, because such matter, being retained for a long time, undergoes coction. He gave the cause of this earlier, saying that, for dysentery, the downward passage is the cause of the quick exit of the excessive matter. On the other hand, for those coughing up matter, the upward direction of this passage is the cause of the slow exit, and for those with matter in their urine, the cause is the heat of that place. If someone does not agree that there is a difference between pus and the 'raw' humor in urine or coughed-up matter or in evacuated matter, this person is in one or the other of two situations. For either he is willingly playing the villain opposed to this teaching, like Erasistratus, claiming that all fevers arise in phlegmatia, or he is a sophist who is unacquainted with the works of this art, whom the ancients correctly termed a *logiatros* (i.e. 'doctor in word only'). For pus differs from the 'raw' humor in color, substance, and smell. And an excretion of the raw humor occurs from the nose and mouth in periods of good and bad health, but the author of this passage above does not bear this in mind.

160-161. He probably said that people in this condition recover "*spontaneously*", as meaning "without our doing anything." For nature will purify them independently. It sets a day for them which is assigned in two ways: one time according to the time of year in which the afore-mentioned excretion happened to start, and the other time extending for one year, but also the short time reaching to forty-five days. Some do not write forty-five, but forty. But I, who have seen many people cleared by nature in this way, know that there are not merely two times for emptying, but a great many. One person is cleansed finally on one assigned day, and another on another, some on the fortieth day, and some extend to an unequal number of months, but there are those who have this persisting throughout the whole year.

161.
Whatever diseases arise suddenly and whose causes are well-known are clearest to prognosticate about. It is necessary that their cure be accomplished by someone opposing the cause of the disease. For in this way the thing in the body which is allowing the disease may be released.

161-162. In this passage he seems to disagree with what is said in the *Aphorisms* (2.19):

The prognoses of severe diseases are not entirely clear, whether of recovery or of death.

And Sabinus himself, when he attempted to resolve this, chattered on, but said nothing reliable. And so did many others who were making an exegesis of this book. And it seems to me that they do not understand what 'suddenly' means. Indeed, they think the term is used for severe diseases which last a short time. But it is not appropriate to use this term in reference to these, but rather, for those diseases having an origin from clear causes, it should refer to one which has arisen in a brief interval of time, as opposed to a longer interval. In these cases, the prediction of what will happen is quite easy, because it is well known what sort of cause there is and how great it is. Those diseases which arise suddenly after a long period of time possess no clear cause of origin, and in the same way their prognosis is not clear. And the immediate causes of diseases are: overheating, chills, sleeplessness, distress, worries, indigestion, sleeping on a hard bed, toil, drunkenness and other such things. For this reason, therefore, he says that "*the cure of such things is accomplished*" by what is opposite to the "*cause*" of the disease, such as cooling if one has been overheated, heating if one has been chilled, resting if weary, exercising more if habitually idle, draining if overfilled, filling if drained, just as he said in the earlier passage which began "*whatever diseases arise from fullness are cured by draining.*"

163.
In the case of those in whose urine there is sand-like material or chalk as sediment, a swollen mass arises at first in the thickest vessel, and it suppurates. Then, as these masses do not quickly break out, chalk grows out of the pus, and is shed through the vessel into the bladder with urine.

If this sort of urine occurred for the reason which he assigns, it would occur when the kidney itself is similarly afflicted, without the large blood vessel being involved. For the excretions in the urine which are so described often occur without swollen masses, when a sufficiently thick or viscous humor, making a slow exit-passage, is dried by the heat of that place and congeals.

In the case of those whose urinations are merely bloody, the blood vessels have suffered.

164. It is not clear what this "*have suffered*" is said in reference to. For it is possible that it means "to be worn out", as these vessels have become weak, and the blood half-cooked, and it allows this to flow easily because of looseness. Or, to judge in another way, it is possible to explain it as "suffering", as apart from "being worn out"; with the kidneys themselves suffering nothing, but the condition existing in the blood vessels alone. Indeed, from such an exegesis it is not clear what sort of condition it is. But it is quite clear that neither Hippocrates nor Polybus would have said 'urinations' (*ouremata*), being able instead to say "*in the case of those whose urines (oura) are bloody.*" For Hippocrates, although he certainly often writes the word 'urines' (*oura*), uses 'urinations' (*ourema*) in no expression. And many other added writings are shown clearly to belong neither to Hippocrates nor to Polybus.

164-165.
In the case of those who have small filaments of flesh in their urinations, which are thick, it must be known that these are from the kidneys.

165. Here he rephrases the *Aphorism*:

in the case of those who have small pieces of flesh, like hair, pass in their urine, this is being excreted from their kidneys. In the case of those with clear urine, who now and again have something like bran carried in the urination, their bladder is flaking.

Again he is rephrasing this *Aphorism*:

in the case of those having something bran-like passing in their urine, which is thick, their bladder is flaking.

166.

Most fevers arise from bile, and there are four specific ones, apart from those arising in separately distinguished ailments. Their names are: the continuous, the quotidian, the tertian, and the quartan. The one called continuous arises from the most abundant and purest bile and it reaches the sharpest crisis, after the shortest period of time. For the body has no time to cool inasmuch as it is heated by great heat. The quotidian, after the continuous, is from the most abundant bile, and finishes more quickly than the others. But it is longer than the continuous, because it arises from less bile and because the body has a rest, while in the continuous fever it rests at no time. The tertian fever is longer than the quotidian and arises from less bile. By however much more time the body rests in the tertian compared to the quotidian – by the same amount is this fever longer lasting than the quotidian. The quartan fevers relate to the others following the same reasoning; they are more long-lasting than the tertian, to the extent that they have a smaller share of the bile which produces heat, and the body takes part in more cooling. This excessive length and tenacity arises for them from black bile. For, of the humors in the body, black bile is the most viscous, and holds its place for the longest space of time. And you will know by this that the quartan fevers have a share in black bile. For men of an age between twenty-five and forty-five are most likely to be afflicted by quartans, and most likely to be afflicted in the autumn. And of all the times of life, this is the one most governed by black bile, and of the seasons, autumn is the most governed. The ones who are afflicted by quartan outside this season and this time of life – it should be known well that their fever will not be lengthy, as long as the man is not suffering from anything else.

167-169. Many of the exegetes, Sabinus among them, seem to me to be affected in a similar way as when a man was ailing with dropsy, and the physician Philotimon thought it appropriate to treat him for hangnail. For it is one of two things: either he does not see how completely ill the patient is, or he does not suppose that treatment is necessary. And thus one must consider that the exegetes either blot out the eye of the mind, or that they suppose that minor complaints require some treatment, but that serious ones do not require assistance. As if wakened from a deep sleep, they perceive the disagreement with Hippocrates made in this passage here, which claims that the 'quotidian' fever lasts less time than the 'tertian', while Hippocrates has clearly said in the first book of the *Epidemics* and in the *Aphorisms* "*the tertian fever comes to crisis the most quickly.*" So they have said that this is not a Hippocratic text, since it clearly says things which are untrue and since it differs from what is written elsewhere by Hippocrates. For in this place alone they understand that the writing which has been appended is false, and disagrees with writings of Hippocrates elsewhere. And if it is in this section alone that they notice that the appended writing is false and disagrees with Hippocrates, then they resemble someone seeing a hangnail and not seeing that the entire body is in a most serious condition.

169-170. Someone who is unaware that the 'quotidian' fever is longer lasting than the 'tertian' fever shows that, on the one hand, he is not skilled in medical works, and, on the other, that he has not constructed a lie due to the madness of someone shameless, but that he was roused by a trusted account, and especially since it seemed to some of the ancients, including Plato, that constant fevers arise from an excess of fire, quotidian from an excess of air, tertian from an excess of water, and quartan from an excess of earth. For a passage from Plato has these very words (*Timaeus* 86a3):

The body suffering from an excess of fire ends up with constant inflammations and fevers; the one suffering from an excess of air, with quotidian fevers; tertian fevers afflict one suffering from an excess of water, on account of it being more sluggish than air and fire; and an excess of earth, the fourth, most sluggish element of all, which, having been purged, hardly ceases in a fourfold period of time, causes quartan fevers.

So if Plato says the most sluggish element, as it is the most settled and least mobile, is cleansed out in a four-fold period of time, it also seemed convincing to differentiate the others from each other by the same analogy, so that it would happen for the next earth-like element, which would be water, that it would be associated with the next closest to a four-fold period, and that the next element again (which is air), would cause the quotidian, and the quickest (which is clearly fire) would cause the continuous fever.

170-171. But more reasonable than this is the account which assigns the reason for the origin of the fevers to the hot element of nature, that is, fire. For it is not good reasoning for the hottest condition to come about from an excess of the cold element in the body. In fact, if it is reasonable that the hot condition comes about through an excess of the hot element, then the fevers differ from each other by differences which should be ascribed to the amount of the cause (i.e. the hot element). And if, indeed, we concede this: that the most constant and hottest fever arises from the most fire, and the next hottest has the second place in amount of fire, and the tertian fever the third place, and quartan fever the fourth, then the dissolution of these fevers will be dependent on the causes: the quickest dissolutions from the hottest fire, the second quickest from the quotidian, the third from the tertian and the fourth from the quartan. So, to the extent of plausibility, these are well said, but the result of the investigation of actual practice disproves the account. And, having nothing reliable to say in his added writing on the anatomy of blood vessels, the one who has fabricated this seems to have been lying not once or twice or three times, but many times entirely, and, in addition, not saying one true thing among these, even by chance.

171-173. It is to be marveled at, with reference to these exegetes, how they object to nothing by the one who wrote all the text after the *On the Nature of Man* up to this point, but now they do object and on this account it seems to them that the entire book is not Hippocratic. Someone may marvel further at Sabinus and most of the exegetes, that they were always praising all these added writings: this thing was written amazingly, according to one man, and that thing miraculously according to another; and another thing divinely according to yet another. And now, suddenly they have forgotten all this, and because of a single conflicting opinion, the book seems to them not to be Hippocratic. But they shift it to Polybus, since they are acquainted with the *Aphorisms* and the first book of the *Epidemics*, but Polybus was not. Polybus, as the student of Hippocrates, must have heard from him many times concerning the differences of fevers, and not a few times must have been acquainted with his writings along with this, and have seen that in illnesses the tertian fever is the quickest to reach a crisis and the quotidian the slowest. For Polybus was not one of those who expounded at Alexandria; not one of those who, having observed nothing yet, afflict the sick person with their skill at guessing, saying nothing sound, and nothing about those things which skillful ones see clearly revealed in illnesses. So the one who has written these things was either such a sophist, or a quack, as seems likely, having appended this lie so that blame might be inflicted on the ancient author. The term, 'continuous' (*sunokhos*) is proof that the added writings are more recent. For in no place does Hippocrates, nor any other ancient writer, call the 'constant' (*sunekhos*) fever 'continuous' (*sunokhos*), just as he does not call 'urines' (*oura*), 'urinations' (*ouremata*), but these are terms of more recent physicians who were ignorant of the ancient wording.

173. Now, leaving these added writings behind, we turn to the *On the Regimen of Good Health*, which they say is a work of Polybus.

www.ingramcontent.com/pod-product-compliance
Lightning Source LLC
Chambersburg PA
CBHW071516210326
41597CB00018B/2784